A CUP OF COFFEE WITH
12 LEADING DENTISTS IN THE UNITED STATES

INSPIRATIONAL SHORT STORIES AND VALUABLE
INSIGHTS INTO A NEW ERA OF DENTISTRY

Elias J. Achey Jr., D.M.D.
Jared M. Van Ittersum, D.D.S.

Rutherford Publishing House
PO Box 969
Ramseur, NC 27316
(336) 824-7012
www.RutherfordPublishingHouse.com

Cover photo: Edyta Pawlowska/Bigstock.com
Cover photo: Christine Langer-Püschel/Bigstock.com

ISBN-10: 0692243267
ISBN-13: 978-0692243268

TABLE OF CONTENTS

ACKNOWLEDGEMENTS vii

INTRODUCTION 1

1 THE TRADITIONAL WAY ISN'T ALWAYS THE RIGHT WAY
by Jared M. Van Ittersum, D.D.S. 3

2 HOW YOU GROW UP DOESN'T MATTER...IT'S THE DREAM
THAT MATTERS
by Elias J. Achey Jr., D.M.D. 33

3 PURDUE FOOTBALL PLAYER TO LVI TRAINED DENTIST
by Charles H. Keever III, D.D.S. 59

4 IT'S THE PEOPLE IN YOUR LIFE THAT MAKE THE DIFFERENCE
by John R. Smelko, D.M.D. 75

5 THIS OLD HOUSE
by Thomas E. Littner, D.D.S. 91

6 THE IMPORTANCE OF A "SERVANT ATTITUDE"
by Ralph D. Beadle, D.M.D. 111

7 ONE OF THIRTEEN CHILDREN
by Timothy Brunacini, D.D.S. 131

8 IV SEDATION CHANGED THE WAY I CAN HELP MY PATIENTS
by Robert G. Ross, D.D.S. 149

9 HOMETOWN BOY RETURNS HOME TO PRACTICE COMPLETE
HEALTH DENTISTRY
by Grant K. Gillish, D.D.S 169

10 PEANUT BUTTER AND JELLY SANDWICHES
by Neeta Chesla, D.D.S..191

11 MY BLUE COLLAR ROOTS KEEP ME GROUNDED
by Nicholas C. Ritzema, D.D.S. 201

12 RETIREMENT DOESN'T MEAN GOODBYE
by Paul R. Voss, D.D.S..213

ACKNOWLEDGEMENTS

We all want to thank our husbands and wives, fathers and mothers, and everybody who has played a role in shaping our lives and our attitudes.

To our dental teams who make it a joy to come into the office and   help shape the future of dentistry – the complete health dental office.

To all the patients we've had the honor of treating, who shaped our understanding of the importance of one's total health. It has been our privilege to serve each and every one of you.

INTRODUCTION

This is a book about relationships and life stories. Every dentist that has been invited to be a part of this book is in an elite category as a clinical dentist. You may already know this as one of their trusted patients; but you may not know the challenges they have faced, the hurdles they have overcome, the joys they have shared, and the life events that have shaped their personality as a dental leader in your community, which in turn shapes your experience in their office.

All of these doctors have one thing in common; they have all joined a group of dentists in an organization called Infinity Dental Partners. Owned and managed by other dentists, this group of doctors are collaborating and growing together to learn from each other's techniques and improve the care they provide. Infinity Dental Partners is pioneering a movement of total health and wellness across the United States by educating patients of a new approach towards dentistry called complete health dentistry.

Taking from all of the new research in the last decade on the mouth-body connection, complete health dentistry is a new era connecting the health of the mouth to the health of other major body systems. As a profession, we are taking a stand against inflammation in the body, and have a unique opportunity to be preventative care leaders in healthcare.

21st Century dentistry no longer represents pain, fear, and inconvenience. It is now centered around education of total body health and establishing relationships that develop trust. Please enjoy these life stories of some of the best dentists in the country, and we hope as a result your connection with your community dentist only strengthens!

Elias J. Achey Jr., D.M.D.

Jared M. Van Ittersum, D.D.S.

Founders
Infinity Dental Partners

1

THE TRADITIONAL WAY ISN'T ALWAYS THE RIGHT WAY

by Jared M. Van Ittersum, D.D.S.

Founder & Partner in Infinity Dental Partners

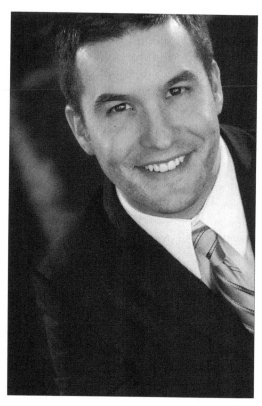

I grew up near a small country town on the west side of Michigan. We lived on a horse farm with my parents and my two older siblings. I loved growing up in the country; I was a dirty little country boy and I didn't even know what MTV was until I was in high school!

I spent as much time as possible outside and even at a young age was required to work hard. I had to work for my allowance in order to purchase the things I wanted. In order for my siblings and I to earn our allowance, my father would create a list of chores for us to do around the farm. Every Sunday night there was a list of about 50 items available to us, such as mowing the lawn (which paid $4), cleaning the barn (which paid $2), doing the dishes (which paid 50 cents) and so on, and he would post the list on the refrigerator. It was left up to the three of us to determine how much we wanted to do and when we wanted to do it. Working for my allowance helped shape my work ethic; it made me appreciate hard work and setting goals at an early age.

I attended Spring Lake High School. Swimming became a passion of mine early on and I swam during a six-year period for three teams. Even though I wasn't tall and lean like some of the better swimmers in school, I was still pretty decent. I ended up going to the State Championships each year during high school and was awarded All State status in my senior year.

I went to the University of Michigan after high school for both undergraduate and dental school and spent a total of seven years in Ann Arbor, Michigan. Suffice it to say, Ann Arbor has a big place in my heart. I took two years off in between undergraduate and dental school because of a unique opportunity that I will share later.

When I was 16 years-old, I had the idea that I wanted to ride my bicycle across the country. I found an event online called the 'GTE Big Ride across America'. It was a charity ride on behalf of The American Lung Association that was held in 1998, and it was the largest cross-country bicycle ride in American history at the time. I received permission from my parents to participate in the event and began a venture that had a profound effect on my life.

In order to participate in the ride you had to raise a minimum amount of money for The American Lung Association. Every participant had one year prior to starting the ride to raise this money and raise awareness for the charity. I started my fundraising with what I thought would be the easy way to raise the money; I created a letter that I sent to hundreds of corporations in West Michigan. In it I explained who I was, what I was doing, and how I was trying to raise money for The American Lung Association.

However, something disappointing happened. I received zero responses. Essentially, every door was slammed in my face. It was coming down to the wire and I only had a few months until the deadline. I had barely raised any money at this point. I had set a goal and was determined to raise the money myself. It wouldn't have been fair to allow kind family members and friends to give me the money in order to participate in the ride.

I had hit a crossroad; I could just give up and say this wasn't meant to be, or change my strategy and my approach to raising the money. I decided to rise to the challenge and took a unique strategy for the remaining 11 weeks. Every day after school I would go door-to-door asking for any available contribution to The American Lung Association from my local community.

I was invited into peoples' homes and I would tell them about myself and what I was doing, I would tell them about The American Lung Association and ask for any donation that they could spare. I literally did this for seven days a week, over the entire 11 week period, and by the end of that time, I had far surpassed the dollar goal I was required to raise in order to participate in the ride.

I learned a monumental lesson from that experience. I learned that, sometimes, the traditional way isn't always the right way. I thought the traditional route would be to solicit contributions from Corporate America because that was what the ride organizers instructed me to do. I felt Corporate America would be excited about helping a 17-year-old raise money for such a worthy cause and would throw money my way. Unfortunately, they didn't, and I had to change my strategy and do something non-traditional.

The other thing that experience taught me was that you shouldn't ever give up. Once you set a goal, no matter what it takes, you have to do everything you can to reach it. It wasn't easy to go out every night, and I had a lot of doors slammed shut on me, and I faced a lot of rejection in those 11 weeks. However, I also met a lot of incredible people along the way.

I also learned to set aside any preconceptions I had about people. I would be invited into homes where I thought the people wouldn't be able to give anything, and they usually ended up being the people who gave the most. The fundraising experience was a very influential part of that event for me. I was awarded the 'Prudential Spirit of Community Award' for the state of Michigan in 1999 for my efforts. This meant I was selected as the number 1 community service volunteer out of 30,000 applicants for the entire state.

A couple of months later the physical journey began. The bicycle ride was from Seattle to Washington D.C., and spread across 48 days. The ride was almost 3,500 miles long and I was the youngest participant of a thousand. I was 17 at the time and the oldest participant was 72 years old. We were like a mobile city moving about 100 miles at a time across the country through the hot summer days.

The event was absolutely indescribable. I was a young man, a high school student, surrounded by hundreds of the most motivated, and some of the most influential, people in the country. One man was the CEO of Time Warner, another was a paraplegic, yet another was 200 lbs. overweight and still able to complete every mile. The ride consisted of participants from all walks of life.

The paraplegic man, whom I became friends with, had a custom-made bicycle on which he had to use a hand crank in order to turn the wheels. Without the use of his legs to pedal the bike, all of the stress was on his arms and his shoulders. He literally rode coast-to-coast using only his arms, hand cranking over every single mile and over every mountain that stood in front of him. It was unbelievable to see someone who had such courage and perseverance ride a bike with only his arms. Believe me when I tell you, it is twice as hard to use your arms rather than your legs to pedal a bicycle; I know because I tried his bike. He never let what some people might think of as a limitation hold him back. There were only 42 of us that were able to bike every single mile and he was one of them. He was just one example of the type of people I was surrounded by on that trip, and the influence they had on my way of thinking was amazing. They showed me that crossing a country as large as the U.S.A. on a bicycle is achievable for anybody.

The trip also showed me what it's like to be around highly motivated people gathered together in a group setting. One of the things I appreciate about our dental organization is that we not only have some of the best dentists in the country, but every one of them is motivated to help provide the highest level of dental care in their community. I feel that some of the power we see in our group practice comes from the collaboration of great minds working towards a common goal, and all of our patients benefit from our collective efforts towards greatness.

I'm very fortunate to be married to my soul mate, Daisy, whom I met in 2008. She is an attorney in Grand Rapids and we had a whirlwind romance. I'm absolutely madly in love with her, and she is a sweetheart to our entire family.

She is Hispanic, from Mexico, and is the only person in her family to ever go to college. Daisy wasn't in a position to get any help, so she worked through undergraduate and law school and made it through to become a successful attorney, all paid for by herself. She has become the shining star of her family.

She was raised in a very difficult situation. Her childhood home was about a 500 sq. ft. house with mud floors and no running water. She had to take showers in the backyard with a hose. There were times when she was growing up, when she had to help her family collect cans from dumpsters in order to put food on the table.

Daisy is a strong partner in our marriage. When you have a strong wife, with her life experiences, you realize that with hard work you can take your life to new places.

I would like to share with you the story about how I got engaged to Daisy. After I graduated from college, I did the whole 'backpack across Europe' thing by myself for six weeks. I backpacked across five countries, either living in a tent or staying at hostels. It was a fantastic adventure. On the trip I went to Italy, and backpacked along the Italian Riviera.

While exploring the Mediterranean, I discovered a magical area called Cinque Terre. The entire area is a historic park and hasn't changed in 200 years. If you were to look at paintings of the Italian coastline, you would often see multi-colored buildings and houses on the hillsides. I can assure you, a good many of the paintings will be of this area.

In Vernazza, a small town within Cinque Terre, there was a little castle on a picturesque point of land looking out to the Mediterranean. I promised myself on this trip that, someday, when I found the woman that I was to marry, I would bring her here to propose. ten years later, I finally found the woman I wanted to spend the rest of my life with.

I asked her parents for their blessing to marry their daughter, and to take her on a trip to Europe to propose to her. I got the green light, so we went on our first vacation together. We toured Europe together traveling to Italy, France and Monaco. I had everything planned out. I even had the ring duct-taped to my leg for four days. I printed out three business cards that said in French, English and Italian that I was carrying an engagement ring, asking to please not ruin the surprise, in case the ring set off the security alarms when going through the airport; luckily it never did.

As we approached Cinque Terre my plan seemed to be working perfectly, until the weather became stormy! Since we were only going to be in this town for a day, I thought it was going to be a disaster. Luckily, just after checking into our hotel, there was a break in the weather that was only due to last for about an hour. So I said, "Honey, let's go and get some nice pictures to send home to the family. It looks like there are some pretty little spots for some great photos."

So we quickly checked in and ran up to the top of this castle point. When we reached the right spot there was a Canadian woman there. My wife is a chatterbox and she started talking to this woman. When we had arrived the sunset was perfect; however, the sunset started fading so I knew I had to get down to business. I was standing behind Daisy and I put the ring above her head and gesticulated the "Shhh" sign to our new-found friend.

It was really incredible because she took the cue, grabbed my camera and said, "Let me take some pictures of you guys." I was able to spin Daisy around and, although I don't really remember what I said, I proposed and she said "Yes". I was lucky and got the whole occasion on camera. I was able to have my dream engagement at sunset on the Mediterranean in this dream spot, and I was lucky enough that she agreed. Our life together has only gotten better from that day forward.

We are very fortunate to have a very beautiful 18-month-old little girl. Her name is Arianna and she was born on May 1, 2012. At the time of writing, we are celebrating the arrival of our second baby girl, Leilani; born on September 9, 2013.

I'm very fortunate to be happily married and I love being a family man. When I became a husband and a father, my priorities changed, and I just love hanging out with my family.

Being a husband and a father also influences everything I do as a business owner and practicing dentist. I try to bring my family values into the way I practice dentistry; how I treat patients, and how I interact with my team members. I always tell my team members, and all the dentists associated with our group, that you spend the same amount of time, if not more, with your team than you do with your family. It's important to make your team feel like family and treat them like family. You need to show them that you have the same honor and respect for them as you have for your family.

In everybody's life there are events that can have a profound impact on them. One such event happened in the two years that I took away from my studies before I started dental school. I was presented with a very unique opportunity to start a business with my father. This was the 'Dot Com' era and we started an internet company called Document Imaging Solutions, Inc., and afterwards another company called EMR, Inc.

We developed a software package that was enterprise-level-software and allowed organizations to become paperless. We even branched into healthcare, where we created paperless medical offices and paperless hospitals. Some of my responsibilities during those two years were to help manage the reseller network. We had over 150 resellers throughout the country that represented our software company. I also developed some of the marketing solutions for getting our software, and our name, into the marketplace.

Very early on, I had the opportunity to work with people from all over the country; clients and resellers, and we really used technology to manage the company. From a small office in West Michigan, we were able to do tele-video marketing through WebEx and put a profound dent in the document imaging industry. Our software was in multiple Fortune 500 companies, as well as in government installations such as the U.S. Naval Command Center.

The list of clients throughout the United States goes on and on, but we were able to grow the business in a way that still allowed us to maintain a family lifestyle, have a lot of fun doing it, and use technology to spread the message and develop our reseller network. It showed me that you can take an idea and grow it nationally more easily than you might think.

Today we use technology to grow Infinity Dental Partners. Although we started out in West Michigan, we're now in eight states and continuing to grow. Using technology provides us the ability to manage our offices without having to be physically at each location.

Starting a 'Dot Com' company, and learning how to manage that company by utilizing technology was the catalyst for the growth of Infinity Dental Partners nationwide. It showed me that, if 10 years ago we could manage 150 resellers all over the country, with the recent improvements in technology we can do it even better today.

Another event that has had a major influence on my life happened in dental school. During my first two years of dental school I helped create what is now known as iTunes U; a product of Apple, Inc. I came up with the idea during my first two weeks of dental school. We could digitally record all of our lectures, and be able to instantly have it organized and put on a range of media devices, but with a focus on iPods. This was at a time when iPods were first released and were becoming a 'hot thing'.

The goal was to be able to record all of our lectures and have them instantly available on our iPod so that when we left the classroom we had that lecture at our fingertips. This allowed us to review our lectures while we were working out, or walking home, or before a test, and have the ability to go back and review salient points that we perhaps hadn't understood during the classroom lecture itself.

After I came up with this idea, we did three pilot studies at the dental school and then we got Apple, Inc. involved. Apple, Inc. got really excited about it and they saw the idea's potential. Apple, Inc. has always been very involved in education so they were a perfect fit. Together we named this iTunes U.

I made several visits to think-tanks at Apple headquarters and had the opportunity to meet most of the executives there. I had some really incredible experiences of collaboration while developing ITunes U. While I was in dental school, I travelled all over the country presenting this concept at some of the larger national education seminars. We were the pioneers in this movement and now iTunes U is in over 300 countries and in thousands of Universities. If you have iTunes on your computer, click on the iTunes U tab and you'll see how powerful it is.

This is one more example of how, through collaboration, you can make great things happen. This was a concept that I envisioned, but I couldn't do it on my own. I collaborated with the dental school and got their IT department involved, and then we brought in one of the largest companies in the world. We collaborated with Apple, Inc. and, together, fine-tuned the concept until it became a reality. This showed me that if you put together the right coalition of people you can make some amazing things happen.

The last experience that has had a profound effect on me was the creation of Infinity Dental Partners. In 2008, shortly after I started practicing dentistry, the economy crashed. I was at a crossroad in my life at which I had to make some changes to be able to support myself and my family, and I was very fortunate to meet my business partner; Elias Achey; the co-founder of Infinity Dental Partners. We started dreaming together.

Once we partnered up, we started purposefully defining our philosophies of practice management and incorporating them into our two offices. When we proved that our philosophies worked, we then believed that it could work in any dental office and we started purchasing more practices, bringing more practices under the umbrella of Infinity Dental Partners.

We began implementing our values and our philosophy of patient care into all of the offices we purchased, even though every single office was different. The doctors at each office are completely different. The teams are completely different, and yet when you put a philosophy into an office that everybody understands and supports, you change the patient experience for the better. Your patients become better educated about their dental care and, in turn, want to take better care of their dental health.

We found that our philosophy towards dental practice management – creating self-empowered teams – took each office to a new standard in how they served their patient family. Everybody from the front desk, to the hygiene department, to the assistants, began working in harmony and sought ways to enhance the patient experience in each office.

Practicing dentistry under our philosophy proved to be enjoyable for us, for our doctors, and for our teams, so we wanted to take it beyond our borders. We believed that it wasn't right to keep what we had discovered to ourselves. We felt that everybody needs to practice the way we practice dentistry. Every patient deserves to experience the care that our patients receive.

We had found something that really hit home for everybody and we wanted to share that with the world. We wanted to grow this concept; of practicing dentistry under our philosophy, beyond our local community. So we started expanding from West Michigan. We started searching for doctors around the country who wanted to take their dentistry and their quality of care to the next level and bring something new to their patients. So we started growing Infinity Dental Partners in other states.

We systematically found the best of the best. We found the best doctors in the country. We don't just let anybody join Infinity Dental Partners. We're an elite group. We injected our philosophy into their offices. We taught their teams how to create a better patient experience. We taught them how to provide better patient education and now, everybody is winning, especially the patients!

One of the things that make us different is that we are a large organization, but we're owned and run by practicing dentists. I understand what it feels like to have a good day and a bad day in our field because I still see patients on a daily basis; I'm not sitting behind a desk crunching numbers and giving out orders. We created a brother-hood and a sisterhood of elite dentists motivated to make their dental offices the forefront leaders in preventative healthcare.

All of my life experiences have helped bring Infinity Dental Partners to where we are now by using the power of collaboration, the power of a coalition, taking motivated individuals, putting them together and really driving a movement and providing complete health dentistry across the country.

What do I mean when I say providing complete health dentistry? To understand this philosophy you must first understand how dentistry has transformed itself over time.

If you look back in history, there have been different phases to dentistry. Prior to World War II, if you had a toothache, you had your tooth extracted. There were plenty of dentists; however, there was really no other way for dentists of bygone eras to treat what we would now consider to be easy fixes, other than by pulling a tooth.

As new research and dental techniques were developed post-World War II, dentists were soon able to insert fillings and had the ability to save a tooth rather than extract it. So, after World War II, dentists began to become more confident in their ability to provide a better service.

Then there was an era in the 1970's when dentists began to understand that a patient's gums were just as important as their teeth. Your gums are the foundation of the house and if the foundation crumbles, the house crumbles with it. There was a lot of research that came about in the '70s regarding the importance of having healthy gums and the implications of periodontal disease, which led to a major era of emphasizing the importance of healthy soft tissues.

Then, computers became more prevalent, there was an era of providing dental offices with technology. It gave us the ability to do same-day crowns and use technology to improve the quality of care within dentistry, and that continues today.

The era we've experienced for the last 20 years has been the era of cosmetic dentistry. Materials used within the field of dentistry have improved and now dentists can insert veneers and bonding, and transform someone's smile. This goes far beyond pain control and improving the function of our teeth. It has been the 'hot thing' in dentistry for a number of years.

Today, we find ourselves in a new era of dentistry, what we call 'complete health dentistry'. There's now enough information to confirm that your mouth talks to your body and your body talks to your mouth. It's not compartmentalized anymore. We no longer only focus on your 28 or your 32 teeth and the gums around it. We now know that there is a very strong communication between your mouth and your body.

Let me provide a couple of examples. We know that inflammation in your mouth leads to inflammation in your body. More specifically we know that active gum disease dumps bacteria and inflammatory byproducts into your body and has a detrimental effect on your heart and your blood vessels. If you have cardiovascular disease and you have rampant periodontal disease, they will feed off of each other. Bacteria and inflammation byproducts exacerbate both conditions. As a healthcare provider, you can't just focus on one or the other; you have to treat them both because your gum disease is making your heart disease worse and vice versa.

Let me give you another example. It's very clear that diabetes has a very strong relationship to periodontal disease. If you have rampant gum disease and your gums end up bleeding, you're sending bacteria and in-flammation by-products through your blood vessels, damaging the vessels and exacerbating your diabetic con-dition. Research has found significant levels of bacteria from the oral cavity embedded in blood vessels all over the body in patients who have active periodontal disease.

I believe this knowledge puts a stronger importance on dentistry in the public's eye than ever before. However, to motivate people to take their dental condition seriously, you have to educate them on these new mouth-body connections. People have to understand the grave systemic consequences of not doing anything with the condition of their mouth. So, in this new era of complete health dentistry, we focus on educating our patients of that oral-systemic connection.

As a dentist, we are positioned in society to offer a tremendous opportunity in preventative health care. Ideally, you see your dentist twice a year, but how often do you see a cardiologist? How often do you see your primary care provider? Personally, I don't see my primary care provider unless something hurts, so I've seen mine twice in the last 10 years, but I see my dentist regularly.

There are a lot of screening aids that we can use as dentists to really be on the forefront of preventative healthcare. I'm working hard to position my industry and the dentists associated with Infinity Dental Partners to be the unsung heroes in healthcare, to be the leaders in preventative healthcare.

We have some incredible tools available to us to screen for systemic disease. Here are just a few examples of what we can do as dentists.

We have devices called VELscopes which allow us to screen for oral cancer at every hygiene appointment and catch it in its very early phase. In fact, we can catch it before it's ever visible to the naked eye. We do this by easily identifying cells and tissues that are changing before they are truly cancer, which allows us to get physicians and oral surgeons involved early on when treatment is easy and stop the problem before it develops into something very bad. Oral cancer is very aggressive. Unfortunately, when you're diagnosed with oral cancer, you have a 5-year prognosis. It's very aggressive in metastasis and spreads to your body very quickly. As dentists, we can catch oral cancer very early with the right technology.

Let me give you another example. We have panoramic radiographs that a patient can be treated with once every year, to five years. This gives us the ability to actually see plaques and calcifications in your carotid arteries. It's an exciting technology because your carotid artery is one of the main arteries to come out of your heart and it's one of the main areas that we see the early onset of heart disease. We're fortunate that in the radiograph we use for dental diagnosis, we also see that area in the neck, giving us the ability to clearly see plaques and calcifications that indicate early stages of heart disease.

I have had dozens of patients in their 50s and 60s who had never seen a cardiologist and were completely asymptomatic. They never knew they had any signs of early cardiovascular disease. By identifying calcifications on the x-rays, I was able to refer them to primary care providers who could evaluate them with a cardiologist. I have had countless cases where the patients had high cholesterol that they never knew they had, and were able to make simple diet changes or get prescribed medication that brought their cholesterol under control.

These patients could have gone another five years and never felt a thing until they had a heart attack. So we may very well help to add many years to these patients' lives. Twenty years ago before we really had a clear understanding of these connections and the technology with which to screen them, dentists were still counting 28 teeth, still focusing on the gums and the teeth, but not really making any connection beyond that.

Our goal at Infinity Dental Partners is to continue to be leaders in dentistry by bringing the oral systemic connection to our patients. We have a responsibility in all of our practices to change patients' lives. Knowing what we know now, we have a duty to change healthcare, and we're changing it. We have positioned ourselves to truly be the premier dental group in all the communities under our umbrella by practicing preventative healthcare and by educating our patients about the oral systemic connection and how dentistry saves lives.

I want to share a little bit about my philosophy about dentistry and the care that our organization provides to our patients. I also want to put into perspective how this philosophy integrates into Infinity Dental Partners.

I'm in a very unique position because I'm still a practicing dentist. I practice full time as a clinical dentist, but also have the responsibility of running an organization with the best dentists in the country. Therefore, it gives me the best of both worlds. As a practicing dentist, I have good days and I have bad days. I have great patient experiences but I also have patients with conditions that present challenges. As I mold the direction of our organization, I use my daily experiences to help guide those decisions and it all boils down to one thing; putting the patient first. Every single decision I make as a leader in Infinity Dental Partners is from the perspective of a practicing dentist and is based around the concept that our patients come first.

When I'm going over a treatment plan with a patient, I tell them, "If you were my brother, my sister, my mom, my dad, my spouse, my uncle, my aunt, my grandmother, my grandfather, this is what I would do for you. If I was sitting in the chair, this is what I would do for myself." I always put the patients first.

Unfortunately, as in any industry, there are people who don't share the same ethos as us, and dentistry has not escaped these few 'bad apples'. In every industry there are times when, regrettably, the patient or customer isn't put first and money or convenience override good values. I have seen scenarios where reputations and trust are lost, and a horrible situation is created when money becomes your number one priority. So every decision that I make is around patient care, and seeing that the patient's interest come first. It's what I teach my team members and everyone associated with Infinity Dental Partners. Everything falls in line when the best interests of your patients are your number one priority.

When a patient visits my office, or indeed, any of our offices, I want the patient experience to be premier. I want them to feel like they're at Disneyland; I want them to have an office tour, I want them to be offered a paraffin hand wax, I want the team to be open, inviting and warm. I want them to know there's a new energy in the dental office and when they leave our office, I want them to talk about our office and their experience. We put a heavy focus on creating an unforgettable experience for our patients.

The other focus we have in our practice's regards premier patient education. Good communication and education are the way to overcome the fear sometimes associated with our profession. With my patients, I want them to know every single thing that's going on when they are in the chair. I talk about every single part of the procedure as I'm performing it. I want them to know what I'm doing and why I'm doing it.

At their new patient exam, I want them to clearly understand what's happening in their mouth and why it's happening. I train my dental hygienists and my assistants to be able to educate patients. We take advantage of technology and abundantly use intraoral cameras to document our findings. A picture is worth a thousand words, and we help create a complete visual understanding of what is happening in the patient's mouth. I want my patients to value the services we provide and I believe that we can create value when they have a clear understanding of what is happening in their mouth, and why it's happening.

We have talked to hundreds of doctors all over the country and what we have found is that the single dental office needs to evolve. It's becoming more difficult for the solo practitioner to practice dentistry, and the benefits to being part of a group practice are undeniable. We've taken a very unique twist on this. As a dentist in Infinity

Dental Partners we treat it very much as a family-friendly, non-corporate environment. To the average patient or team member, you wouldn't know that your dentist is a part of Infinity Dental Partners. We want everybody to feel like it's a private practice, and we work hard to maintain that 'private practice look and feel'. That's how I make my patients in my existing practice feel, and I believe it's extremely important to maintain the individual identity of every office.

There are, however, a lot of benefits that can be gained from joining a group. There are a lot of pearls of wisdom and tools that we can learn from each other. We believe in collaboration within our group of dentists, and we're always learning from each other. There are tips and tricks that I've learned from all of my dentists, and I have incorporated them into my daily practice to provide better care. Dentists who are in their own stand-alone clinic are on an island. There are other dentists in town that are looked upon as colleagues, but you commonly keep your best pearls close, as ultimately your colleagues are also your direct competition. It's what sets you apart and makes you unique in your community. But when you're a part of Infinity Dental Partners, everybody benefits from your wisdom. We are all here to help each other succeed. I give out all of my pearls – everything that I know makes for better care - creating a really unique learning environment that has made our dentists even more elite.

Our team members also have their own collaborative groups in order to learn from each other, and they are always improving themselves. We have philosophy coaches come in to help train team members in how to create a better patient experience; how to have a philosophy of better education; of treating patients as number one, and how to make every single patient feel like that every single time they come in.

So we found that you can still have the look, feel and integrity of a private practice, but you can get the benefits of a larger group. That's where I see the future of dentistry. I see the future becoming collaborations and coalitions. I see the development of more group practices. I see our organization growing as people see the benefits because it really is what we call the quadruple win. We win as an organization, the dentists that join us win, the team members that are part of that practice win, but most importantly the patients win because they directly benefit from the improvements. I guarantee that the thousands of patients who are under the umbrella of our organization are receiving better patient care than before their offices joined our organization.

There are going to be a lot of changes occurring in the healthcare industry within the next couple of years. As we move towards a universal healthcare approach there will be good and bad things involved, but overall one thing that is very clear is that preventative healthcare is going be of the utmost importance in this revolution in healthcare. As I've mentioned before, we have an opportunity as dentists and as a dental industry to be the leaders in that movement. Oral systemic care and the complete health dentistry model really allow us to make dentistry the screening point for healthcare. Again, you see your dentist twice a year but you really don't see other healthcare providers unless something stands out. We have a responsibility as dentists to use that to our advantage and use what we know about the systemic connection to screen and prevent major systemic disease in our country. We must all unite to educate the public so that we are the pioneers and the shining stars in this national preventative healthcare movement.

2

HOW YOU GROW UP DOESN'T MATTER... IT'S THE DREAM THAT MATTERS

by Elias J. Achey Jr., D.M.D.

Founder & Partner in Infinity Dental Partners

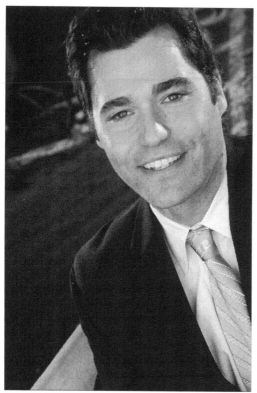

I grew up in San Bernardino, California, and we were constantly moving. My mom was addicted to drugs, and life was like a roller coaster, up and down. My dad has been a millionaire three times, and he lost it all three times.

One time stands out: when I was in first grade and my dad lost it all. We didn't have a place to live, and we ended up in a shelter that was just like a big warehouse. That was a really weird point in my life, but living through those difficult times now empowers me, and the memories help push me forward to the life I live today.

While in this low-income housing, my dad got his real estate license and started buying and selling property. Things got a little bit better for us, and we were able to move out of there to a better area of California.

While growing up, I had a couple of best friends. We would play baseball in the street, and we had our own BMX bikes and Oakleys when they first came out. We had our own little BMX gang. We'd spend our days outside and jump our bikes all day long, just having a good time.

Unfortunately, that's when my mom started doing drugs. Without her supervision, I stopped going to school because I enjoyed riding bikes more than I enjoyed going to school. I would pretend to go, but instead, I'd get on my bike and take off. Then I'd meet my friends after they got out of school.

It was during that time that I started getting involved with gangs, and I started going down the wrong road. I never did drugs, but I started affiliating with the wrong crowd. It was a blessing in disguise that my dad lost his company and we moved from California to Alabama.

My dad had a client in Alabama who agreed to work with my dad to develop a property that he owned. So at that point, my dad just closed the doors, packed everything up, and we drove to Alabama in an '89 Ford Probe. To this day, I remember the car being packed with all our stuff, as well as me, my mom, and my little dog, Oreo. We went from this booming metropolitan area of San Bernardino to a town with two traffic lights in Alabama.

I feel that move helped me to become a man and not behave like a kid. I started learning manners, and I started learning about life. I went back to school, and I had to get tutored because I hadn't developed the education I needed, having skipped school in California.

It was during this period of my life that I actually discovered what dentistry was all about and decided that I wanted to become a dentist. I remember the event like it was yesterday. I was in eighth grade, and my cousin was getting married. He was in dental school, and he sat with me for about two hours. We talked about dentistry and about life in general. I saw how happy he was, and I wanted just a piece of what he had. I just wanted to experience the happiness he was experiencing.

After that talk, I knew I wanted to be a dentist, and I started making As and Bs. I went to high school at Enterprise High School in Alabama in the small town we moved to from California. It was a pretty cool high school, and I have a lot of fond memories there. When we first moved, it took a while to get into the "good old boy" network, but high school was fun and I had a good time. I made a lot of close friends.

After high school, I went to junior college for a year, and then on to the University of Alabama. My strategy was to go to a school that had a dental school. Even before I was accepted, I wanted to go to the dental school and learn as much as I could about dentistry. So I went to the University of Alabama, Birmingham, and majored in Biology and Chemistry. After graduation, I went straight into dental school.

To this day, I believe that dentistry saved my life, and I feel honored to be where I am right now in my life. I'm living beyond my wildest dreams.

Today, my partner, Jared Van Ittersum, and I own twelve dental practices in eight different states across the country. So when you look back at where I was and what has happened, it is almost unbelievable. I am now surrounded with incredibly talented and highly motivated people, and it's almost hard to take it all in. It's hard to feel like you deserve something like that.

If you don't mind me getting a little philosophical here, we all have major events that shape our lives as we move forward. Besides the talk I had with my cousin that influenced me to turn my life around and become a dentist, there are several other factors that had an impact over the years.

One was the inability to be able to hang out with my father and to have a stable home life. That has really impacted my life, driving me to make sure that I provide a very stable home and life for my children. I remember one time my dad took me out fishing. I cherished that moment even then, and I remember similar moments with my father that I cherish today.

I always wanted to have a great family life, so I was willing to do whatever it took to get it. I think that's why dentistry has remained so attractive to me. Throughout the years, I've been able to set my own hours, have my own company, and be my own boss. It has always stuck with me that dentistry has limitless potential.

A part of Michigan influenced my life. I have an aunt and uncle, Lynn and Buck Boersma, who lived on Spring Lake in Michigan, and it was my heaven on earth growing up. It was the place that I would go to that was the life I always dreamed of. I remember we would sit out on the porch and Aunt Lynn would come out with some fresh fruit. Or we would be in the lake swimming, and when she came out, we would run up to the porch, eat, and then go back into the lake. We'd wake up in the morning, go out on the dock, look at the bass and the sun fish, and life was good. Why wouldn't it be, if all you have to do is fish, play in the water, run up to the house to eat, and then do it all over again?

Just being able to experience that life and see the relationship that my Aunt Lynn and my Uncle Buck had was incredible. They were high school sweethearts, and to this day, even after being married for thirty-six years, they still hug and kiss each other like they're in high school. By experiencing that life, I knew that it could be possible for anyone, including me. I knew that a strong marriage between two people who cared deeply for one another could be possible, and wanting that life really drove me to become a success. It was my dream life, the house on a lake with a beautiful wife and a wonderful family.

I now have a beautiful wife, Anne Claire, a beautiful nineteen-month-old daughter, Margot, and an awesome five-month-old son named after my dad, Elias. My wife comes from modest means; she was born and raised in a small house in a small town in Mississippi.

We're building our dream house in Nunica, MI as I'm writing this chapter. Having a stable home and growing up in one place is the one thing that I always wanted for my kids, as well as for myself. Now I can provide that lifestyle for my children, and that really is very special for me.

Graduating from a dental school was also a major event in my life that has had a profound impact on me. To be quite honest, I never thought I was smart enough to even get into dental school, let alone get out of dental school. I think that while growing up, I didn't have the self confidence that a young adult should have. I just didn't feel like I could do it, and when I did graduate from dental school, it proved to me that I was smart enough and that I could accomplish my dreams and desires.

Another such event was getting accepted to the cross-country cycling team. That was the first time I ever got accepted to anything that I really wanted to do. This happened at a time when I was trying to get into dental school, and I had just been denied. When I got onto the team, I felt that I was finally part of something big. It allowed me to ride my bike across the United States with a team to benefit people with disabilities.

While I was on that cross-country ride, there was one moment that stands out in my memory and shows me that kindness can change someone's life. It was in California. We had stopped at a home for people with disabilities, and there was a lady with cerebral palsy who had been abandoned by her parents. This family found out about it, adopted her, and gave her a computer to communicate with. To this day, I remember walking up to her and putting my hand on her shoulder, and she smiled so big. I had never seen a smile this big before. She was smiling from ear to ear, and that's an under-statement. She had such a huge smile and I remember that moment touching me deeply. Even though we stopped every day at a home for people with disabilities, this one girl sticks out in my mind because all it took was a touch on her shoulder to make her happy.

That cross-country bike trip had a profound impact on me. It changed my perspective on life. It made me be thankful and appreciative of all the things we take for granted, such as just being able to walk, ride a bike, or take a deep breath and breathe naturally. From that moment with the girl, I learned that it isn't always the big things in life that leave lasting memories, but it can be something as simple as a touch on the shoulder, or simply giving someone an authentic smile.

I tell our dental team to show people that you're happy to see them and smile. You never know when a smile can change a life.

I remember the day I found out I was accepted to dental school. Most of the people had received their acceptance letters in December, and this was May. It was my third year of trying to get into dental school, and I hadn't heard anything one way or the other.

One day, I walked out of the house and went to the mailbox. There still wasn't a letter from the school in the box. At that time, literally everybody who applied was either getting a decline or an acceptance letter. So I called the admissions board at the school and asked, "I'm just wondering what's going on in my application?"

The girl on the other end of the phone replied, "Yeah, I think you were accepted. But let me check to make sure." And I remember my heart racing, like I felt that I was going to have a heart attack. Time stopped and I literally thought to myself, *Oh my God, this is really happening. Is this really happening? Please come back and say that I really got accepted!* She came back and said, "Yeah, I have the letter right here. We're gonna send this out. Yeah, you got accepted to dental school."

When I hung up the phone, I ran up and down the hall of the house I was renting. I was screaming and crying. I fell on my knees, and I was so excited that I sat there and prayed, literally, for an hour, just thanking God for getting me into dental school. I was so excited. I couldn't wait to tell everybody.

I called my dad and I said, "Dad, where are you?" He was driving, and I said, "Dad, you need to pull over." So he said okay and pulled over to the side of the road. I said, "Dad, I just got accepted into dental school!" and he screamed and cried. It was just an amazing event in my life and for my family, and the next week I got my acceptance letter from the University of Alabama. Later, the dean of admissions told me that "they had a little argument over who was going to call me because everybody was so excited to let me know that I was accepted into dental school, because they knew how hard I had tried to get in." I have to tell you, that was one of the best moments of my life.

Another huge event for me was meeting Gary Kadi. I had just purchased the practice in Whitehall, and I was lost. I didn't know anything about insurance, managing people, or anything else business related. All I knew about was practicing dentistry.

I have always battled with feeling like I deserve what I have. I had a very low deserve level and Gary Kadi was really able to coach me into becoming a stronger leader and believing in myself. I was able to learn some of his philosophies that helped me understand that life won't give you what you deserve, but what you feel you deserve.

Learning to have a healthy deserve level was a game changer for me, and I've since discovered that it's one of the pieces of the puzzle to achieve a successful life. In fact, I believe that it eventually led to Jared becoming my partner, and everything that has come from our partnership. It was like planting a seed, and from that one seed a whole garden would grow. Having Jared show up in my life was something that I never saw coming. Jared and I have come to discover how much we think alike, and we have become like brothers. From our relationship a whole garden of dental practices has grown.

For you to understand how I care for my patients, it's important that you understand my philosophy about dentistry.

At first, I got into dentistry because you never have to sell anything. You get to set your own hours, and you get to make good money. Over time, my philosophy has changed. I've discovered that you have to make it all about your patients and your team because without a winning team, everybody loses. You lose. Your family loses at home because you're losing at work, and you bring that home with you. The patients lose because they aren't getting the treatment that they deserve. They deserve to be in a good environment right when they walk in; they deserve to hear laughter in the office.

So, my philosophy changed from centering around what kind of dentistry I want to do to focusing on what of kind of person I want to be. So it's not all about cosmetics or about technology. To me, it's all about how I can make my team happy, and in turn, how my patient is benefiting from the team being happy.

One of my beliefs is that you have to be able to change the lives of your team members so that they change the lives of the patients walking in the front door. You can have integrity as a doctor, but your patients don't know that. They learn about you by hearing what is being said in that exam room after you leave.

We can't expect excellent and energetic service to be routinely provided to our patients unless our team members (those with patient contact and those in support functions), who provide that exceptional service, are themselves engaged in an active personal pursuit of growth and excellence.

Our belief is that whether, they be doctors, hygienists, assistants, or front office team members, their purpose is to become the best version of themselves.

It's almost like the saying, "You build it and they will come." Well, if you build a positive environment, the patients will come, the money will come, the happiness will come, and you will be able to change the world through dentistry one patient at a time. That's my philosophy now.

I know that there will be doctors who read this book and wonder how Infinity Dental Partners came about. So this is what happened.

My cousin had a satellite office-- in other words, a second office at a different location. So from early in my career, I started thinking: wouldn't it be nice to be able to have multiple locations, and what could happen if you have a group-type practice?

With a group practice, everybody could learn and benefit from each other. So I came out of school and had the idea that I wanted to have multiple practices. The problem was that dentistry had become so corporate, and when I was in dental school, everybody was talking about the issues with corporate dentistry. It was failing the patient miserably.

When Jared and I became partners and talked about our futures, I said, "Jared, wouldn't it be sweet if we could buy multiple practices but not make it 'corporate?'" And it was from those conversations with Jared that Infinity Dental Partners was born. We both felt the same way: we never wanted Infinity Dental Partners to be seen as "corporate dentistry."

We decided that in order to isolate ourselves from the image of corporate dentistry, we had to be invisible to the outside world. We felt that it was important to maintain the identity of the office that we were purchasing.

We decided that we didn't want to be simply one of the best of the best. We wanted to be the only ones who do what we do.

When we first started defining the idea of expanding our group practice, we wanted to create an environment in which everybody in the office had fun, from the team to the doctors. What we realized was that a lot of the doctors we talked to weren't having fun practicing dentistry anymore. The burden of having to manage the practice was exhausting and frustrating for many of them. We decided that, if we could eliminate the burden of management from the doctors so that they could focus on dentistry, it would remove a huge amount of stress from their lives and let them focus on what they loved to do.

We also knew that each dental office had its own DNA, and we didn't want to change that. We wanted to respect the practices' uniqueness; after all, in most practices the team has been together for years and developed their own way of doing things. So the challenge would be to manage the practice in a way that recognized this fact yet brought in systems that improved workflow, incorporated a higher level of patient education than most practices had ever seen, and made the office a fun place to work.

We wanted a group practice that would change people's lives for the better. So we started researching management companies and extracted the best parts of what each one was doing. Then we began implementing them into our practices to test each of the systems. If it didn't work as we anticipated that it would, we threw it out and kept only those parts that supported our goals. If it had a positive effect on our team members, our doctors, and our patients, we kept it and worked to improve it.

We developed Infinity Dental Partners into this group practice that is non-corporate and changes the lives of everybody associated with it. We are taking the best of everything we can find in dentistry, everything that has a positive impact on our teams', doctors', and patients' lives, and incorporating these systems, strategies, and philosophies into every office that becomes part of our organization. It works, and for Jared and me, it's been a truly humbling experience to see how we can impact so many lives in such a positive way.

I mentioned earlier in the chapter that Gary Kadi has had a big influence on me and my philosophy about dentistry, and here's why. Every year Gary Kadi invites about 15-20 doctors to a think tank about dentistry, and I was invited to go to Cancun, Mexico at the Ritz Carlton. For me it was a life-changing experience because we focused on where we wanted to take dentistry. In other words, we got to redefine ourselves as dentists and how we felt the industry should serve and care for its patients.

The topic the first day was: What is dentistry known as? It's stinky... It's smelly... It takes time out of the patient's day. It's not the "hip" medical profession.

Being a dentist is not a "hip" thing to do. It's the profession with the highest suicide rate.

Then the second day, we talked about what we want to make dentistry known for. We wanted to be known as a profession that is changing lives. We wanted the profession to get the respect that it deserves. We wanted dentists to be educating patients on the mouth-to-body connection so that our patients could become healthier. We wanted to be the profession that is known to be very giving and life changing.

On the final day of this think tank, we had the responsibility of formulating a statement that would become our compass for how we wanted to move into the next era of dentistry. We came up with "pioneering total health and wellness for all."

When you think of a pioneer, you think of a guy climbing over a mountain to get to the Promised Land. We're climbing this mountain of misconception of dentistry. In communities across the nation and in the medical field, people don't realize how connected the mouth is to the body. If we're going to change dentistry, we have to edu-cate the public about this connection. After five years, this is beginning to happen, but there is still a lot of work to do.

If you picked up and are reading this book, I want to take a moment to provide you with some critical information you need to know.

There are endless studies showing how tooth loss leads to many years lost from your lifespan. There are studies showing the relationship of problems in your mouth to diabetes and low birth weight.

Knowing how the mouth is connected to the body, dentists can now catch problems in the operatory. Today we have the ability to take a pictographic image of your head and your neck, and in the digital image we can see the plaque that may be in your carotid arteries. We can educate you on what could happen if this is left untreated, and refer you to your cardiologist so that they can treat you. The bottom line is that there is a link between high quality of life and a healthy mouth.

Currently, Jared and I are talking about creating schools for health and wellness, where Infinity Dental Partner doctors can teach other doctors how to educate their patients effectively on total health. The goal is that the patient understands why a doctor is recommending a particular treatment plan and is motivated to accept treatment.

I see Infinity Dental Partners as limitless. I fail to understand why a doctor wouldn't want to become part of

Infinity Dental Partners. Currently, a doctor has to worry about the burden of management, wherein he is the CEO, the CFO, the marketing director, and the human relations manager. He is all these people, yet he says he wants to give the best care to his patients. We have found that a doctor performs his best when he is free of these responsibilities and can focus 100% on his patient.

A doctor has the responsibility of the operations, or the nuts and bolts of his practice, and he also has a responsibility to his patients. If you're so stressed out throughout the day about all the management stuff, how will your mind be 100% on that patient? What Infinity Dental Partners is doing for their doctors is taking the management burden off the doctor so they can focus on the patient.

So to me, it doesn't make sense not to become part of Infinity Dental Partners, where a dentist can become part of a movement to change dentistry and take it in the direction that it needs to go. That direction allows doctors to provide the highest level of patient care, keeping in mind the systemic relationship between the mouth and the body, to be able to focus 100% of your time on your patients and not have to deal with all the management issues. And finally, to become the best version of himself or herself because they interact with other doctors who are there to support their efforts and share their knowledge with one another.

Let me share what I believe is the biggest difference between Infinity Dental Partners and what we know as the typical model of corporate dentistry: I would say it is our philosophy. Our philosophy is that if you change the lives of your team members, in turn you're going to change the lives of your patients. Furthermore, if you change the lives of the patients then you will change the world.

Corporate dentistry oftentimes will fire much of the staff who has been with a practice for a long time because their salaries tend to be higher than what they can hire a younger person for. We don't do that. We value older employees and understand that they have often built relationships with the patients in the practice. Why would we want to let go of someone who has a strong relation-ship, many times spanning decades, with a patient? Corporate dentistry is driven by the numbers and typically tells its doctors and hygienists that they have to hit certain numbers in order to keep their jobs. We don't do that either. We won't tell a doctor that he has to shorten the amount of time that he's going to be with his patients so that we can hit our goal that day. Our focus is one of providing the highest quality of dental care for our patients, educating them on how important it is to keep their mouths healthy, and retaining them as patients for their lifetimes.

We want everyone in our offices to connect with their patients and know what matters to each one individually. Patients are not just numbers to us; they are people who we know and see in the communities that we serve.

Furthermore, we don't come in and slap a sign on the front of your building that says "Infinity Dental Partners." We're not into mass marketing on TV. We are not into micromanaging by numbers. We believe in a philosophy of caring for our patients, our teams, and our doctors. If you believe in this philosophy, and you believe in a movement to change dentistry to a higher standard, everything will take care of itself. What we have found is that this belief has proven itself to hold true with all of our practices.

One of the things that Jared and I believe is that it is important to find ways to give back to each of the communities we live in. One of the ways we found to do that is to hold a Free Dental Day.

The first Free Dental Day we ever held I will remember until the day I die. The day of the Free Dental Day, Jared and I were walking up to the office at five o'clock in the morning.

There was a line out of the parking lot. When I say line, I mean there were probably two hundred and fifty people lined up in the front of the building, and they were cheering us. They were clapping. They were just so excited that we were providing free dentistry to them because they simply couldn't afford it due to their life circumstances. We were so taken back because it was raining, and it was cold, and they'd been standing in line for hours. Some of them had been there since five o'clock the night before.

All we saw were smiles on their faces, showing just how happy everybody was to be there. We were so tired coming into the office at that hour, but by the time we walked through the front door we were stoked. You kind of get this adrenalin rush, and the team was excited too. The thrill of such an appreciative crowd of people was infectious.

I remember starting that day when this young girl walked in and sat in the chair. She must have been in her 20s or early 30s. She was noticeably shivering. We literally went out, got a blanket, and put it on her. We actually were worried about hypothermia because she had been sitting in this rain for so long. I noticed that she had a plastic bracelet on her wrist and I said, "That looks like a hospital bracelet. Did something happen?" She said, "Yes. I was in the hospital for a tooth infection, when somebody in the hospital told me that White Lake Family Dentistry is doing a free dental day. When I heard that, I checked myself out of the hospital without the permission of my physician. He said that I needed to stay there and get IV antibiotics." She said, "I know I need to see a dentist, but I didn't have any money to pay for the dentistry."

She was sitting there telling me this story with her eyes closed. Then I numbed her, and I could see her shoulders noticeably drop into the chair. Her whole body just went limp because that was the point I got her out of pain. I then removed the tooth, and she was crying. I was crying. Everybody was crying. Everybody was just very, very touched by the moment. And that's when I knew, right there, that the whole event was worth all the work that it took to make it happen.

That event told Jared and me that we had to do this every year in every one of our offices. Although it is just one of the ways we try to give back to the community, the fact is, we receive more than we ever gave to these people. We are all thankful that we are in a profession that lets us have such an impact on people's lives.

When I look at the direction in which dentistry is moving, it worries me. Without Infinity Dental Partners, I believe that dentistry is moving toward corporate dentistry, where it becomes about bonuses, and it becomes about how many people you can stuff into the chair during one day. It's about how many patients come through the front door. There's no doubt about it: that's the current path the profession is taking.

Jared and I have created Infinity Dental Partners to protect our profession from that ideology. The biggest difference is that we see corporate dentistry as dollar-driven, and Infinity Dental Partners' philosophy is patient-focused.

We want to consider the patients' personal motivators. What drives that patient to get up in the morning? If you don't know the most critical values of your patient, then you don't know your patient.

There is little doubt that dentistry is changing, and I believe that dentists are going to be on the front line of healthcare. It's almost to the point where the insurance companies are demanding an oral exam before a patient goes in for any type of surgery. We are beginning to see the public understand how important your mouth is to quality of life.

It's important to remember that almost everybody has teeth, and therefore, everybody needs a dentist. That gives dentists an opportunity to reach people and touch them in a way that can change their lives. We should never forget that. We should never forget how special dentistry is.

Like many dentists, I've been on a mission trip, and in the middle of a desert seen fifty people who have walked over a hundred miles to have a tooth removed. I've seen people line up two hundred and fifty deep to see us on our Free Dental Days. When you experience these events, you see just how important dentistry is to people all over the world, not just here in the United States. It drives home just how valuable our profession is.

3

PURDUE FOOTBALL PLAYER TO LVI TRAINED DENTIST

by Charles H. Keever III, D.D.S.

Muskegon, Michigan

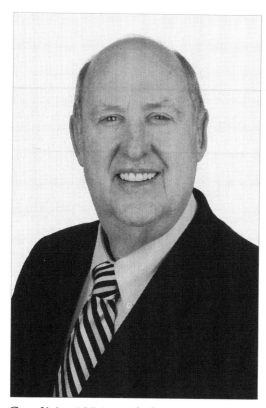

Growing up in Indianapolis, my life was filled with sports - everything you can think of, including baseball, basketball, and football. I played a lot of golf and enjoyed every minute of it. My siblings and I did everything together. In 1952, I was the firstborn, followed by twins Kurt and Candi in 1954, and then our sister Kim in 1956. We were all close, played a lot of sports together, and had a lot of fun. We did everything together, especially Kurt and me.

During my senior year in high school, I was accepted at the United States Naval Academy. I really wanted to be a carrier pilot because I loved to fly. When I went in for my final physical, it turned out that I had astigmatism in my left eye. That washed me out of flight school; you could be a navigator, but you couldn't be a pilot. That was disappointing, because I had my nomination and everything. At the same time, Purdue was calling me to play football for them, and they were a top 10 school. When I decided not to go to the Naval Academy, then everything went in the other direction. That was probably my biggest turning point as a kid. Life directed me to Purdue, then to dental school, instead of being in the armed forces. I graduated from Pike High School in 1970 and played all the sports: baseball, basketball, football, and track.

I went to Purdue as a walk-on football player and majored in pre-dentistry. Basically, when you're playing football, your life revolves around the sport. You don't get much extra time. My biggest priority was to make sure I made it to every class, so I started at 7:30 every morning and got done at about 2:30 to get to practice. In college, I was either in the football stadium or in class.

One of my best games against Michigan was a home game during my senior year. I had a couple of quarterback sacks in the first half, and when I came out the second half, I was double teamed on every single play for the rest of the game. They didn't like me in their backfield.

Then I had another really good game. We were at Minneapolis, playing Minnesota, and I still remember that game to this day. It was 8 degrees above zero; I had on long underwear and a sweatshirt, and we were still cold. I swear, when we hit each other, you thought your body was going to break in half. I had 11 tackles and a couple of assists by the end of the game, which was on national TV. I had about 50 phone calls from everybody when I got back home. My dad got calls from all over the country because that was the time when they only had one game on TV. It was a national game, so that was great, especially for my father.

That was a great time because I was in Pi Kappa Phi Fraternity House, and my parents made it to all the home games. One of my family's close neighbors had a motor home. They would come up for the home games and basically feed the entire fraternity house before the game. My parents would cook all kinds of stuff, and my brothers at the house would make room for a special parking spot for the motor home every Saturday. They all got fed really well.

On my mother's side, my grandfather and great grandfather were both dentists. My grandfather graduated from the Indiana Dental College in 1919. On my father's side, my grandfather Keever is on the first pictures of the football team that are hanging in the Assembly Hall. From 1916 to 1917, he played two years as a fullback at Indiana before he went on to medical school, so I feel like I followed in his footsteps.

He was Marion County Coroner in Indianapolis during the 1930s. For 50 years, he was also the physician at the Indiana School for the Blind. During a big discussion with both of them, my grandfather Keever told me, "If you really want to have a family life, be a dentist." I saw that, as a physician, his life was never his own. He couldn't get away from the telephone no matter what he did. He was always getting phone calls, 24/7. So I took his advice and went the dental school route. Besides the two most impactful experiences in my life (my first marriage and having children), graduating from dental school in Indiana runs a close third in terms of life impact.

What got me to Michigan was my first wife, who was originally from the Boston area of the East Coast. She did not want to live in Indianapolis. I didn't want to live in Boston, so we settled and lived in Michigan. I had taken family vacations as a kid in the Holland area, but when I got out of dental school, five new dentists (competitors) had just moved there. Up north, I went into practice with Dr. Jim Hegedus, who was looking for an associate in Muskegon. Of course, graduating from dental school was a big step, as it was my life's career at that point. After graduation, I searched for a truly good learning experience and found that with Dr. Hegedus. He was my mentor, and I really enjoyed my time with him.

After going through a divorce, I met my second wife, Carrie, who has been a wonderful influence on me, calming my nerves and keeping me in line. Carrie and I were bumped off of a flight together. She was coming back from Kansas City, and I was coming back from a TMJ course in San Francisco. We both flew into Detroit, and the weather was really bad. The weather in Muskegon had gotten worse, so they had to add extra fuel onto the plane to deal with the cold. This caused the plane to be overweight, so they asked for volunteers to take another flight. I was one of the volunteers and so was Carrie. We actually met getting our tickets for the next flight. The airline gave us a dinner voucher. There was actually another girl too, and the three of us went together to Cheers Bar in Detroit at the airport and had dinner. Right after dinner, since I had a Northwest World Club membership, I took them to the World Club and we got free drinks. Carrie and I just started talking, and we really hit it off.

Carrie knows how to talk to me to keep my blood pressure down. That is important because dentistry is a stressful job. She knows how to handle me. We've been married for 12 years now. The family is expanding. At the moment, we each have two girls and five grand-children (three grandsons and two granddaughters), and another on the way.

My daughter, Kelly, and her husband Mike live in North Muskegon. She's the only one who's close, and she has our granddaughter Addison. My other daughter, Kristy, and her husband John live in Grand Haven.

My stepdaughter, Amy, and her husband John, as well as my other stepdaughter, Allison, and her husband Adam, live in Normal, Illinois. It's hard to get down and see them all the time.

Being a grandparent is just a lot more fun because you can wind up the grandkids and send them home. It is funny when they come over to grandpa and grandma's house. They don't want to leave, imagine that! We've been giving them treats, but we're trying to watch our food intake a little bit. The kids do have a lot of fun with everything – pool, lake, and the like.

I've always been a person who strives to be the best; you're not an athlete without having some drive to excel. When I got out of dental school, I wanted to get into doing some orthodontics, so I went to United States Dental Institute for a number of years. Towards the end of my training, they started courses on removable orthodontic appliances. I wanted to learn more, so I started taking a lot of courses from Dr. John Whitsitt, and he was great. He was my first introduction into the world of temporomandibular joint (TMJ) diagnoses and treatments because it followed orthodontics. At one of the advance courses I attended, I met Dr. Larry Front. He was an orthodontist in Bethesda, Maryland, who had started a TMJ study group, which I joined. In that study group, we had some really great teachers. Among them was Dr. Janet Travell, a great lady who was former President Kennedy's personal physician while he was in the White House.

At a lot of our courses, she taught us trigger point injections, and the myofascial pain and dysfunction part of treating TMJ problems. I wish I could have plugged into her knowledge base. She was brilliant. After that study group, at that point in time, I did everything when I was treating TMJ patients, or going through Phase II of treating TMJ. I was pretty much doing all orthodontics.

Since that's too time-consuming, I started looking for a way to treat TMJ patients successfully without having to do it entirely by orthodontic methods. That's how I came across Dr. Bill Dickerson and the Las Vegas Institute (LVI) camp around 1998. LVI is a conglomeration of all phases of dentistry: endodontics, periodontics, crown and bridge restoration, and a lot of orthodontics. Basically, all phases of general dentistry are taught at LVI, with the emphasis on treating patients with pain and TMJ. More recently, the focus is on treating patients' sleep apnea and obstructive sleep apnea.

My actual philosophy concerning dentistry and patient care is total body health treatment. That has been my philosophy since I started. It's not just treating the teeth, but helping to make sure that every patient is in the best possible shape. I have been trying to integrate a lot of our medical knowledge with dental knowledge, and getting people referred to the doctors who can handle the medical aspects of their health if they are beyond my scope. It's about total body health and welfare, and that sounds pretty good. This philosophy is what I've been practicing for 35 years.

I decided to become associated with Infinity Dental Partners when we were recruiting Jared to be my associate while he was still in dental school. I was recruiting Jared with the understanding that when he came on board, after he had been in practice a few years, we would reverse roles. I was getting just a little tired of dealing with the management aspects of dentistry, and of dealing with the government. It's just too time consuming and crazy. I had found the right partner in Jared, and I felt very comfortable with him coming in, being my associate, and taking over for me. Now I get to go home at 5:00 o'clock instead of staying late at the office.

There actually was a break in the relationship because of economic conditions; the great depression hit Michigan very hard. There wasn't enough business to keep everybody busy when the economy collapsed. Elias was doing well in Whitehall, and it made sense for Jared to go to Whitehall and work with him. We said that as soon as the economic conditions improved we could do things together. Once the economy started improving in

Michigan, I was the first acquisition of Infinity Dental Partners. I am extremely happy that I took the leap of faith and sold to Jared and Elias.

Mainly, I was completely burned out on dealing with all the management aspects of the practice. Management pressure was starting to create a lot of health problems. As soon as Jared and Elias started taking over the management aspect, I could relax and just do the things that I wanted to do. Man, my life sure improved - a lot. My wife, Carrie, could really see an immediate change. It was like a great weight had been lifted off of my shoulders because I felt so much responsibility to all the girls in the office. I was starting to have some real heart problems, and if I went down, I was worried that these girls would be out of a job.

It was like I became a new person once that weight was lifted off of my shoulders. Now, I can go home and relax, not having to worry about the office until I come back in the morning. I can give my patients a lot more time, and treat my patients more effectively because I'm really with them; there's no need to worry about this other stuff going on behind the scenes.

Without all the distractions of being a multi-tasker, I'm able to focus strictly on patient care. For example, I no longer have to deal with all the girls in the office or worry about who is or isn't getting paid, and the other office distractions. I can say, "Hey, colleagues, go talk to the boss upstairs. I'm out of it. I have no say in that decision." It's kind of a good feeling.

As with anything, the hardest part was giving up control. You're used to being the man in charge and now you're not, so you just have to get used to the new routine. Well, I've been adapting really well. I'm enjoying myself. My wife is enjoying me being home on time for dinner every night, instead of getting home at 7:00 or 7:30.

I now have the ability to go on vacation without worrying about who's paying the bills. That's been a really big point because I just had my first long vacation in 35 years. I was gone for 17 days. That's the longest I've ever had off in the 35 years since I graduated. I told them not to call me unless the place was burning down - and even then you can't call anyway. Knowing that Dr. De Boer and everybody else were here to take care of things was very relaxing. I think that is one of the biggest points for anybody looking at what we do here in Infinity Dental Partners. Probably one of my biggest plusses is selling the practice and just being able to cut back a little bit and enjoy life, having your own life instead of letting the office run it.

Although I sold the practice, Jared and Elias still ask for my input. They always ask me, "Okay, what about this person? Meet him and see what you think." So you can still have input as to who's here and who's not here. They rely on the doctors in the practice to keep them informed. If the doctors are not getting along with one person in a practice, it's not going to flourish, and there will be ongoing problems. You try and get things worked out just like in any practice, but the doctors still have input. I like the fact that you're not 100% out of operations. You're still the main person working and producing, so you have to be efficient. You have input into the people who are working, and are training those who are working with you. I've enjoyed having the chance to do some training with the new associates, especially in occlusion and some other minor facets of TMJ. I've especially enjoyed teaching people about some aspects of occlusion. It's not taught extensively enough in dental school, in my opinion.

Occlusion is a term that means "how the teeth are supposed to fit together." It's like gears – the teeth should be fitting together just like finely engineered gears. Whether they're not meshing perfectly or there are points of conflict that make the teeth hit each other, that's occlusion. Ideally, everything is working smoothly and efficiently and causing no pain.

Most of my office team has been with me for over 20 years. Any time you bring in new management, there are always changes. People like some of the changes but not others. Dealing with the staff was causing grief for me because they were my friends and family. They weren't employees anymore, they were family, and you know how difficult it is to deal with family members when things go awry. Before I sold the practice to Infinity Dental Partners, it reached a point where I found myself making decisions based more on emotion than on sound business practices. I came to the conclusion that I couldn't separate the business from my personal attachment to my team. When that happens, it's time to get out before the emotional upheaval breaks you. When you have a problem with personnel, it's like going through a divorce. It's very, very emotional, and the way my health was going, it was darn near killing me. Between that and the government, that's why I sold the practice, so I could get my life back together.

I see the future of dentistry following the medical model, meaning, going into the bigger groups or joining a group practice. For the next 10 to 15 years, only a few individual dentists, I believe, will be working by themselves. You're going to have to be in groups, if for no other reason, than to cope with all the regulations. You have to be able to amortize the cost of those regulations over a wider group to be able to make a profit. That's why you see very few physicians who have individual practices. They all work for the hospitals right now.

I think dentistry is going to become a bigger part of personal healthcare. We are starting to see more and more evidence of things in the mouth causing medical problems. There was a big article in Science Daily just last week about how mouth bacteria can cause colorectal cancer. The mouth has microbes that have been linked to colorectal cancer. There are proven links between periodontal disease in the mouth, and diabetes. I think those medical links are going to increase as our knowledge base increases. I would say to people: "What I tell you today is for today, what I tell you tomorrow will probably be different." It's just like the materials I used five years ago; I no longer use them today. There's always something new. There's always knowledge. Our knowledge base is increasing at exponential rates, and that will never stop. The knowledge that we have today is going be outdated tomorrow. So, I have to date everything I say.

That has been unbelievably true in my TMJ practice. Just in the last two years, the way we take bites has changed dramatically and increased our knowledge base. One thing I especially love about Las Vegas Institute (LVI) is that it's a living laboratory - tens of thousands of patients have been treated out there. We take our own patients out there to work on, and when I do a full mouth reconstruction, it's not the only case going on. They're doing 10 or 12 at a time because we've got 10 or 12 different dentists in that course. Over time, they're refining our techniques in every class.

I was taking a course on my K7, which is what I use to measure electromyograms, three-dimensional jaw movement, et cetera. I was taking an interpretation course for those scans. Four months later I was again at LVI because I was finishing up a full-mouth case in the clinic. I finished early and stepped in on the scan interpretation course that I had just completed three months before. It was so funny. There were unbelievable amounts of new information they were teaching, and the change was drastic for such a short three-month period. That's why I go out there a couple of times a year. There's always something new, every single time. It's not just a little thing that's new; it's usually something that's pretty significant that you need to know.

Through the experience of having several dentists within the group, I've enjoyed the benefit of having access to one another and the freedom to share information. A lone practitioner, unless he goes to LVI or someplace like that, just doesn't get that same type of input. We need to have our own forum, though I'm actually feeling a little overwhelmed by the amount of information. This morning, I was caught up on my LVI forum, and now just a few hours later, there are 89 emails to read. Unfortunately, if you're out and about, and if you're not getting really good CE, then you have to go the forum route – it's the only way to learn.

I see the role of Infinity Dental Partners as that of a group providing excellent care. Everybody, including me, has a lot of knowledge that they should be able to share. There's always more than one way to treat a case. Like on the LVI forum, "What would you do in this case?" "I've got this problem, how would you treat it?" And if everybody can go on there and say, "Okay, I've got this idea or that idea," you could formulate the ideal way to proceed. That's what we do in the forum. You'll sometimes get 10 to 15 different ways to treat the same thing, or warnings on what to watch for. You'll have guys say "Look out for this, I had this happen to me" or "Watch out for this and make sure this doesn't happen," and you really learn a lot.

I have learned a lot. It's like going to school. I'm here at least an hour a day, and it's like I have an hour of continuing education every single day. You're not getting credit for it, but it's fantastic.

4

IT'S THE PEOPLE IN YOUR LIFE THAT MAKE THE DIFFERENCE

by John R. Smelko, D.M.D.
Punxsutawney, PA

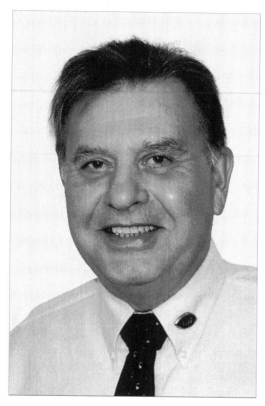

I was born and raised in the small town of Punxsutawney in Western Pennsylvania. Punxsutawney was a great place to grow up and had an excellent school system. My family and I lived right in the center of town so my parents did not need a car and did not have one until I was ten years old. We walked everywhere, to school, to church, to the grocery store and to sports events.

I was fortunate to be born into a terrific family. My mom and dad worked hard and managed to raise six children. Funding twenty-seven years of college, they were always there to support us. My dad taught us about the significance of education. Four of my sisters graduated from the Indiana University of Pennsylvania. The fifth sister elected not to go to college and is the toughest, hard-working one of the bunch. She was my office manager for sixteen years and was very efficient. In my mind, she earned an MBA of life.

Surprisingly, my love of sports is one of the reasons I am a dentist today. When I was thirteen years old, I missed a dental appointment to play a baseball game. Sure enough, a couple of months later I had a heck of a toothache. I was able to get in to see my dentist. I remember sitting in the dental chair preparing myself for treatment. I was in pain! He began drilling and I jumped. He hit the nerve, so he made the decision to extract the tooth. With six children, he figured my parents were unable to afford to save the tooth. I went home biting on bloody gauze and the tooth wrapped in a tissue and handed it to my mom. I think she was shocked. I saved that tooth and now have an implant in place. Doc was a great man, and to this day I credit him with the choice I made to become a dentist. He practiced in Punxsutawney for fifty-five years and God willing I will beat that record.

Growing up, I played a different sport each season and most of my friends are guys I played some sort of sports with. It didn't matter what it was, I played it, and I was fortunate to be a member of some great teams, and coached by two Hall of Fame coaches.

In 1960, our Little League baseball team played in the State Championship but lost to Levittown, Pennsylvania.

Levittown went on to win the Little League World Series. During 1963, our basketball team was undefeated. On November 11, 1963 we played our last game and finished 10 to 0. Our basketball team made it to the State Quarter Finals.

My 10th grade English teacher and basketball coach was Chuck Daily. I played on his final high school team when I was a sophomore. He went on to coach the "Dream Team." He won gold medals and the World Championship for the Detroit Pistons. He is in the National Basketball Association Hall of Fame.

I also had a high school football coach who had a huge impact on my life. His name was Jack Hart, and he is in the Pennsylvania Scholastic Coaches Hall of Fame. Coach Hart helped get my acceptance into Bordentown Military Institute, which, at that time, was no easy task. I was just an average kid, but he made the phone calls to the right people and, because of him, I got a chance to grab the ball and run with it. Being around these great people motivated me to want to further my education and succeed.

It is obvious, I live for sports and I had a great teacher, my dad. From an early age, he became a fanatic about Notre Dame, especially their football program. He often told his story about how it all began. His dad took him at age 10 on a train from Punxsutawney to Pittsburgh to watch Pitt vs. Notre Dame in 1928. After the game, my grandpa and dad stood outside the Notre Dame locker room, awaiting Knute Rockne. When Knute came out, my grandpa walked over introduced himself, and asked Coach Rockne if he would shake my dad's hand. At that moment, my dad became a lifelong Notre Dame fan. He and my mom attended every football game for twenty-five years. On October 2nd of 1992, Notre Dame was playing Stanford. My dad was not well, but he would not miss this game. Notre Dame was up 16 to 0. Stanford made a comeback and beat Notre Dame 33-16. It was very hot that day and after the game, my dad suffered a stroke on his way to his car. He always said he'd die in South Bend, and I'll be darned if he wasn't right. When my dad passed away I purchased the 50-yard line seats that he had held on to for thirty years. The year after his death, I went to a game at Notre Dame and I buried in the end zone a tooth I extracted for him years before. I like to think that made my dad laugh.

After graduating high school, I went to Bordentown Military Institute thanks to Coach Hart. Bordentown provided me with the necessary tools I needed to increase my academic ability since I spent most of my high school career focusing on school sports. While at Bordentown, I played football and baseball for two years. I played in the position of defensive back. I was on the kick off team as a special plays team player. Of all the sports I played, I enjoyed football most. Baseball was fun, but football was more intense and you have to put your game face on if you plan to succeed.

Like many other military schools, Bordentown became used less and less and is no longer operational. However, I met many great friends and athletes during my time there. Bobby Bell, my teammate at Bordentown Military Institute, was the first round draft choice for the Lions. My roommate, Charlie Hall, was the Packer's third round draft choice. One of our offensive tacklers, Stan Walters, played twelve years for the Eagles, and now he provides the radio commentary for them. Additionally, Floyd Little was a running back at Bordentown and he is in both the College Hall of Fame and NFL Hall of Fame. Norman Swarzkopf, Vietnam War veteran, commander of the U.S. Central Command, and four-star general in the U.S. Army was also a graduate of Bordentown.

When deciding a profession to pursue, I knew I wanted to help people. Being able to help others was, and still is, most important to me. I knew that dentistry would allow me to do that.

After Bordentown Military Institute, I was awarded a scholarship to the University of Pittsburgh for Army ROTC. I also attended the University of Pittsburgh's School of Dental Medicine. On May 19, 1974, I graduated from the University of Pittsburgh, School of Dental

Medicine. This was a major accomplishment for me because I completed an eight-year doctoral program in seven years. The graduation ceremony took place in Pittsburgh at the illustrious Carnegie Musical Hall. After the ceremony, my dad shook my hand and said, "Good job, son. There were times I didn't think you had it in you." It was a truly meaningful moment for me.

Soon after graduation I began practicing dentistry. My intention was to work for the benefit of others. I was fortunate enough that word of my practice spread, and word-of-mouth is the best advertising you can have. After 40 years of practice this remains true.

As an adult, there have been three major events that have influenced my life: graduating from dental school, getting married, and becoming a father. Marrying Loretta was really significant because I never thought I'd find my ideal match. I was pretty specific in what I wanted, and when I met Loretta, I knew she was the one.

My best friend, from childhood, introduced me to Loretta on a blind date. It was the summer of 1976. He had been trying to set us up on a blind date for a couple of months, but she was an emergency room nurse and had to cancel our date three times. On the fourth occasion, we had a date set for 7 o'clock, meeting in the town of Dubois. I was a hundred miles away in Pittsburgh. It was about 3 o'clock in the afternoon, and I was saying to myself that I should cancel the date, just out of spite. Fortunately, I thought, "What the heck, I'm not doing anything anyway. I might as well go to Dubois." So I made the trip to meet her, and the rest is history. We met on August 20, 1976 and we're still married, now with three children.

Becoming a father was something I took very seriously. I have three children, 1 daughter and 2 sons. Both Loretta and I had wonderful parents, and I wanted to emulate them. I always wanted to put my children first.

Adrianne is my firstborn. After high school, she attended to Lehigh University majoring in Journalism, then onto Rhode Island School for Design, which is one of top fine arts schools in the world. Adrianne also wrote and published a book entitled, *For a Moment.* She resides in Santa Cruz, California.

My eldest son, Sebastian, attended Carnegie Mellon University after high school. He played four sports teams in high school and college football. After his undergraduate studies, Sebastian moved on to Law school at the University of Valparaiso. He now lives and works as an attorney in Indianapolis, Indiana. He is married to a wonderful young lady, Heather, who is also an attorney.

My youngest son, Alex, attended the University of Vermont and then onto Pittsburgh Art Institute to study photography. He is a self-made chef and musician. At any family gathering Alex is the chef, photographer and entertainer. He resides in Denver, Colorado.

At this point in time, my kids are healthy and lead good lives, something I couldn't be happier about. I am not a grandfather yet, but I am looking forward to having grandchildren while I'm still young.

Providing individualized and compassionate care means that you have to take the time to really listen to your patients. When I got my doctorate degree at the age of twenty-six, I had a talk with my dentist. He told me something I never forgot. "Listen to your patients, because they will tell you what you need to know in order to provide them with compassionate care." So, I sit with my patients and I listen. I want to know about their families and their interests. If you take the time to get to know and understand your patients, they're going to trust you.

My team and I have continued to provide our patients with the compassionate care just like I would want my family to receive. My purpose and vision as a dental care provider in a rural community is to share with my patients the value of a healthy mouth and how it affects total wellness.

Every morning, on the way to the office, I turn my car radio off and say a little prayer, "God, guide me today because I need help in making these decisions and in carrying out the treatment successfully." Sometimes you do a job, look at it, and know it's not perfect. Sometimes you have to stop and do it over again to be satisfied with your work. I take pride in what I do. I want my patients to be able to walk into any dental office, have the dentist look at his or her teeth, and see that I did a good job. "Integrity" and "tenacity", two words my dad lived by and I strive to live by.

I know there will be some dentists who will read this book who will want to know how I became involved with Infinity Dental Partners. It began with a letter in the mail. It didn't have a return address on it and I normally wouldn't even have bothered reading it. Fortunately, Loretta read it. The letter that came from Infinity Dental Partners was only a couple of paragraphs long, but it struck a chord with me. We decided to take action, and Loretta emailed them right away. We began to learn more about Infinity Dental Partners. I liked the idea of two young guys trying to do something to help the dental industry, and I wanted to be part of their effort.

The more we learned about Infinity's philosophy, the more we felt it was the right decision. We attended their West Michigan Summit meeting. We were so enthused after the summit that it made the whole journey worthwhile. Following the meeting, we were required to go through a very thorough step-by-step procedure.

We are excited about being part of Infinity Dental Partners and having the opportunity to work with two young, forward-thinking guys. As a solo practitioner I never had a partner in dentistry. It has been a great experience getting to know Jared and Elias who are such good people and talented dentists for such a young age.

When Jared and Elias spoke at the West Michigan Summit, it motivated me when I saw their vision. I was impressed with their demeanor and the way they complemented each other. I was also happy to learn that we shared similar interests, including a passion for the outdoors, sports and a love of our families. For dentists considering teaming up with Infinity Dental Partners, who may wonder if Jared and Elias are genuine, I can say without any hesitation that they are the real deal. They are highly regarded dentists with a lot of integrity, and I'd be proud to call either one of them my son. They represent their families, universities, and profession admirably. With their quality care and the use of technology, Infinity Dental Partners are working to make dentistry a better industry, and helping people to better understand total health dentistry.

Infinity Dental Partners is driven by a sound philosophy. As dentists, we see the effect the mouth has on the body as a whole, and there is more and more information being released to increase public awareness. The philosophy behind complete health dentistry is that the mouth affects everything. If you want a healthy body, you need a healthy mouth, because you can't have one without the other.

The venture with Infinity is an intimate, personal experience that makes my dental team and my patients feel like they are part of something.....something very important....complete health. My patients and my community are seeing that dental care impacts overall health.

Infinity Dental Partners has implemented a formal process where all the dentists are able to interact with each other. We share our experiences and we all learn from each other. I have discovered that Infinity and I are on the same page concerning patient care. I am more effective in educating our patients about the recommended treatment. When a patient leaves my office, they leave with a customized profile of how to obtain the best dental health. This includes a treatment plan with intraoral pictures so they can see what needs to be done and why it's important to their overall health.

Becoming part of Infinity Dental Partners is like a breath of fresh air. Not only is it great to be involved with a couple of young guys working to improve the dental profession, it has also given me a new sense of purpose. I always knew about the healthy mouth/healthy body connection, but Infinity has the whole concept put together, making it easier for me to communicate this to my patients and for them to comprehend.

I really take pride in telling my patients that I have a support system with Infinity and how my office was chosen first out of a thousand dental offices in rural Pennsylvania and in New York. Knowing that some-body else has recognized the hard work that I, along with my team members, have been doing all of these years, it fills me with pride. When I share this with my patients, it energizes me.

Infinity Dental Partners can also be credited with improving my quality of life by providing me with a sense of obligation to me. When I am out on the front lines preaching the significance of a healthy mouth and body, I better practice what I preach. I am now making it a point to get myself in much better physical shape. I focus on my eating habits and physique. I'm busy, but I challenge myself to find the time to exercise. I regularly work out on an elliptical machine. It's my own program for self-improvement. My patients have seen the difference. If they haven't seen me for six months, they pay me compliments and ask what I am doing differently. Infinity Dental Partners has motivated me to start thinking about my own health as part of the equation. If I'm healthier, I can better serve my patients. I am happier and healthier since I joined Infinity Dental Partners. I smile when I think of Dr. Achey and Dr. Van Ittersum, and I am so blessed to have met them.

Anyone considering joining Infinity Dental Partners should be prepared to make significant changes. If I were to sit down over a cup of coffee with a fortunate prospective dental office, I would tell them that it is well worth it. Dentists often do not want to change or try new things. If they join Infinity Dental Partners, they will become a part of a high-quality system, and they must be willing to make adjustments in order to work within that system. It will take some change, but I'll tell you, I would do it again. Nothing good is easy; you have to be ready to adapt to the guidelines of Infinity Dental Partners. It's not difficult as long as you go in with an open mind and a lot of energy, because that's what it's going to take.

It has been a long and eventful journey to reach this point. I built my life on top of the foundation my parents laid for me. I stuck by my values and worked hard. I focus on my family and put integrity and heart into everything I do. I am a lifetime member of American Dental Association,

The Pennsylvania Dental Association, University of Pittsburgh Alumni Association and a Century Club Member of the University of Notre Dame. Along the way, I received guidance and inspiration, from family, friends, my dentist, coaches and my team. I would not be where I am today without them. Taking this step to join Infinity Dental Partners gives me a greater sense of purpose and new found energy. I am proud of where I come from, where I am, and where my path is taking me.

5

THIS OLD HOUSE

by Thomas E. Littner, D.D.S.
Middletown, New York

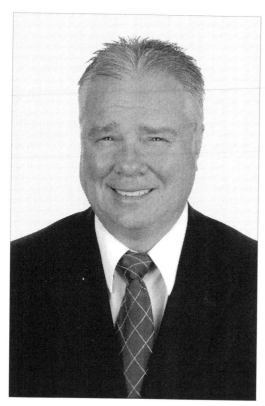

I grew up in Middletown, New York, in a blue-collar family of two children - my sister and I. I made a lot of good friends at Middletown High School, and loved to play soccer. My father was a hard-working correctional officer, while my mother was a stay-at-home mom most of the time. She had a big influence on our early years. My sister was a cheerleader in high school and we got along well growing up.

Our somewhat sheltered lives had a basic routine. Once in a while, we would go on vacation. We were raised without extravagance and lived a good, basic, healthy life with a loving family. We visited our aunts and uncles and focused on family activities throughout our childhood.

My mother had various jobs while I was growing up, one of which was as a legal secretary. (She could type faster than a speeding bullet.) At one time, she had a job as a receptionist at a dental office. She saw the dynamics within the dental office and discussed her observations at home. She said to my sister, "You know Jeanne, you could be a hygienist. It looks like a wonderful job earning decent money; you could be independent." She kept saying that dentistry was a nice profession, and that opened my eyes to it as a possible career choice.

I always enjoyed studying the sciences (especially biology) and math. I thought that in order to enter into the field of dentistry, knowledge of these scientific subjects would be required. Luckily, that was the area of my education that I enjoyed the most. I did a lot of early research while picking a potential career. I looked through big, thick, employment manuals and researched the requirements of employment within different sectors. I also considered becoming a forest ranger because I like science, but when I looked at the job opportunity for forest rangers as well as the potential income, I decided against the idea. While looking at dentistry as a profession, I realized that the dentist owns the business, work hours are good, and it's possible to earn a decent income. It seemed that dentistry would be a good fit for me, since I also liked helping people. So I decided to enter the field.

During high school, I made some good friends. I also had a girlfriend, whom I had dated for a number of years during high school, and through my time at college.

After being away at college, I would come home to Middletown and visit her, and we would do all our studies and homework together. Traveling back and forth from college to Middletown, I felt like I was getting pulled on both ends. When I got accepted into dental school, I told her, "I'm going to dental school in Washington, D.C. If we're going to continue our relationship, you're going to have to come with me."

However, she had other plans. After so many years of being together, the whole relationship came to an end. I thank God for that now, because I was able to focus on my work at dental school.

I met Theresa, my wife, after returning to Middletown to practice as a dentist. We were at orientation at the psychiatric hospital, to train for our positions. I showed up in a suit and tie, she was in her uniform, and we just started chatting. Our joke today is that we're both crazy because we first met at the psychiatric center. It was a great first meeting and things progressed from there.

I am so thrilled to be married to her. We have three children and our life continues to be great. Marrying Theresa was the biggest event in my life and I feel truly blessed by God. Tyler is now 25, Cosette is 22 and Blaise is 19.

At 56 years old, I have been practicing dentistry for 30 years. During those 30 years, I have encountered a number of situations regarding team members and patient situations. I would often jokingly say, "I could really write a book. You wouldn't believe all of these different things that have happened."

You don't often hear of this happening anymore, but I started my practice from scratch. I came home to Middletown thinking that starting from scratch would be the best approach to become a dentist in Middletown, since my parents knew a lot of people in the community. I also knew a lot of people, having grown up here. Luckily, beginning work at a psychiatric hospital allowed me to concentrate on starting my practice on evenings and Saturdays in a space rented from another dentist in town. From then on, I've slowly but surely built up my own practice.

The house that I grew up in also played a part in my work. We had moved when I was 5 years old, and we rented out the "other house" to college students, because the college is right down the street. After starting my dental practice in Middletown, I bought the house from my parents and renovated the ground floor into my dental practice; I lived upstairs. Buying my childhood home is important to me, and gives me a sense of having roots within the community that I'm still living in today.

Over the years, it's gone through renovations a number of times as the practice continues to grow.

I strive to keep my business at a professional level at all times. We do our best to have fun as a team, but the bottom line is that the practice exists for the patient. If it weren't for our patients, we wouldn't be here. I'm the type of person who will never forget his roots, and I'm thrilled about being able to help the people in my hometown community. Living and working in this community is what I enjoy. I serve the people in my community with respect, because I want the best for my patients. Also, since I'm from Middletown, the business is personal. I'm aware that my personal reputation is at stake as well as my professional reputation.

To be at the cutting edge of dentistry, I do a lot of reading and research, and I'm very interested in health and wellness. I'm on staff at our local Orange Regional Medical Center and I often interact with medical doctors. Over the years, I've worn a sleeping aid in order to combat snoring, and I feel the need to pass along the benefits of that technology to others with similar problems. After years of using the sleeping aid, I increasingly realized the link between general health and dentistry. The more research I did, the more I realized that patients' medications are intertwined with their over-all health and dental well-being. This included patients dealing with diabetes, periodontal disease, high blood pressure, stroke, heart disease, obesity, and sleep apnea.

I'm also on the Cancer Tumor Board along with medical doctors. When someone needs cancer radiation treatment, they first come to my office for screening. I check for active infections in their mouths. If there is an infection, I either remove the tooth or do whatever is necessary to get them stabilized, so they can proceed with their medical care. I get a lot of personal satisfaction from helping my patients feel better and healthier.

For example, one of my female patients had a front tooth that was severely discolored. It was obvious that she had somehow knocked it at some point in the past. During our examination I discovered that there was an abscess in the tooth and an active infection was in process. It was not swollen, but it was a chronic condition. When I discovered that the tooth was abscessed, I said, "we've got to do something to get back your beautiful smile. We have to get rid of this infection." After a root canal, I sent her home with antibiotics, as that is the usual treatment for this condition. A few weeks later she came back for another appointment, sat in my chair and said, "You know what, Dr. Littner, you have literally changed my life."

I was amazed - and grateful! Although my work is always the best it can be, only a few patients have told me that over the years, and it was really nice to hear. I said, "Really, you feel that much different?" She answered, "You have no idea. Over the last few years, I've been feeling horrible. I've been feeling really tired, and I've only been able to bail ten bales of hay a day." (I thought that was pretty good, I don't know if I could even do that). We talked for a long while and she said, "I feel so much better after you helped me with the infection. I have so much more energy. I can't believe how much more energy I have." I then asked, "So, how many bales of hay can you bale now?" She answered, "Believe it or not, I can bale 70 hay bales now." That story stays with me. There is no doubt that there is a relationship between someone's dental health and their overall health.

Since becoming involved with Infinity Dental Partners, I feel like I am even more integrated with the medical community and the overall wellness of my patients. I have always put my patients' needs first and provided them with the same level of care that I would provide to my Mom and Dad. Over the years, I have found that by treating patients in this way, they have faith and believe in you and accept the treatment that you feel is best for them.

Since I have practiced for years the concept of total patient health, when I associated myself with Infinity Dental Partners, it was a great fit. I always strive to provide the best quality of dental care for my patients, and that is the

Infinity philosophy as well. Giving patients the ideal treatment will make them feel the best that they can feel, and look the best that they can look. We offer our patients a full treatment plan from the smallest of fillings to implant dentistry, dentures, oral surgery, root canal treatment, etc. Our philosophy is that complete and compassionate care makes our patients happy. When patients are treated to an ideal level of health, this starts a good cycle of reciprocation. As a dentist, you feel stronger about your abilities and the patient will listen to you because you feel more confident in yourself. Treating our patients to be as healthy as possible works well both ways.

When patients first come to us, we gather all of a patient's medical information and establish a warm, friendly relationship to make them feel comfortable. We also examine the information that they give us about their medical health history. We then review their medical history with them, and have a conversation about how the health of their mouth impacts the health of their whole body. By doing this, trust is established, and the patient doesn't wonder why we are asking medical questions that a doctor would usually ask.

Over the years I've had people ask, "Why do I need to give you this information, since you're just a dentist?" Since I am a doctor, I explain to the patient, "Well, this medicine you're taking makes your mouth dry. If your mouth is dry all the time, what happens to your teeth and your gums and your bone, do your teeth decay?" Their common response is, "I don't know." When I explain to them that this information affects how I treat them with regards to their dental care, I usually hear, "Nobody ever explained that to me before." Going through this process establishes a relationship of trust between you and your patient; they realize how much you care about their health.

It's an educational process for every patient. Over the years, I've learned that you need to educate everybody. When you do that, you're on your way to making sure that they're okay, physically and mentally. Their medical history may include a list of medicines for high blood pressure, cancer treatments, or anti-depressants. Though all of this is important and provides us a wealth of information, it doesn't mean much unless we sit with them and make sure that they understand the systemic relationship between their medical history and their mouth. Our patients see that we care and are different from other dentists they might have visited in the past.

So I've begun to ask myself, "What am I going to do with the rest of my life?" As far as the transition process is concerned, that is the biggest decision that a private practice doctor needs to make. There are a lot of questions: "How am I going to end my practice? What will be my legacy? How am I going to get paid? What am I going to do about retirement? Do I have enough money for retirement?" All of these question tend to go through everybody's head as they approach my age. At 56, people say to me, "Oh, you're young," but do you know what? It takes time to make these transitions; it pays to start thinking through these issues as soon as possible.

Working with Infinity Dental Partners is helping me to make decisions faster, but it still takes time. Without their help, thinking about transitioning would certainly have been more difficult. First, I would have had to find and train an associate. Then I would have had to ask myself, "Will this associate have any available financing?" Dentists fresh out of dental school will certainly have difficulty raising the amount of money needed to buy a practice. I'm not sure that they would be able do it after considering the amount of debt they have coming out of school, and banks' general lack of desire to lend money.

To learn more about available transitioning options, I attended several seminars, because it was the biggest question that I was facing. At one seminar, the speaker told everyone, "Quit looking for a magic bullet." He said, "Do all of you guys want to retire? Get off your fanny and build your practice. If you want to be able to transition out of your practice, you had better build it up so you can sell it. You need to get in those new patients." He focused on what we had to do in order to build up the practice, bring in the new patients, and get busy. It was like he was talking to me and saying, "Don't even think of transitioning at this time."

He wanted us to read a book entitled, <u>The Science of Getting Rich, The Science of Being Well, and The Science of Being Great</u>, written by Wallace Wattles. I purchased the book and it changed my life completely. I recommend that every single person read that book. It really explains the law of attraction. It talks about how you should live your life based on the following principles: gratitude, health, wellness, helping others, what you think about will come about, and just do the right thing.

I said to myself, "What am I going to do about preparing for a transition?" My building, at the time, was a little bit too small. So, I decided to take a leap of faith and increase the size of my building. My goal was to get enough operatories within my building, and then get an associate to join me, so that I could start working the process to eventually sell to the associate. We had only three operatories at that time. I kept studying this book and praying. I was almost obsessed with it because I thought I needed to prepare for my later years.

I finished the office construction and it turned out beautifully. I was blessed with having a great contractor. We worked hard on the project, and didn't close the office for a single day during the construction phase. It was amazing! The contractor was that good. I scheduled my open house on Flag Day. As soon as I had done that, I got a letter from Randy Van Ittersum about the possibility of becoming involved with Infinity Dental Partners, and the process began. I sent them my financial statements and we had a number of interviews. I traveled to Michigan, and got a lot of people involved: lawyers, accountants, my wife, and friends.

It was a difficult process because I couldn't involve any of my team members, and I couldn't talk to anybody about it. It was very secretive and it was really, really gut-wrenching. I was hoping and praying that the association with Infinity Dental Partners would come about. At the same time, I tried to prepare myself in the event that it wouldn't happen. I always felt like this association had the potential to be something really great.

Then, suddenly, it happened. My practice became the New York office for Infinity Dental Partners. Since that time we've been forging ahead, adjusting, changing, and building on the principles I've always pursued. If you want it to happen, it will happen, but nothing is easy. If you want to be successful in anything, it requires hard work. That's the stage that we're at now. It's now been three quarters of a year since we became associated with Infinity Dental Partners and things are going well.

I'm completing this chapter of the book while on vacation in Michigan. When I was planning to take some time off, I realized that what I really wanted was to get out to Michigan again. It was just something I wanted to do; to see everybody again, reconnect, and meet others who are also part of Infinity Dental Partners, like their book-keeper. I felt (and still feel) that I am really integrating into the organization. I wanted to get out and meet some people who we interact with but never get to meet in person. It's not because I am forced to socialize on a business level, or anything of the sort. It's just because it's the right thing to do.

Traveling to Spring Lake, Michigan, and initially meeting Jared and Elias was great. Jared and Elias know what they're doing, and quite frankly, they have great business acumen and people sense. I have found that they do the right thing with everyone. Their main role is to organize and maintain the practices in order that they have a good flow, good integration, and good relationships with their patients. They do everything they can to insure that everyone is on the same page and can effectively communicate with each other. I wanted to continue to socialize with these guys because they were a lot of fun and, in my opinion, they are living life correctly. Today they are at the office, doing an extreme makeover, laminates and all. They're integrating their services with other medical doctors and companies in the area so that they can change people's lives. The bottom line is they are helping patients to achieve total wellness, healthy bodies, and healthy mouths. They do what it takes to make these things happen.

I'm just so happy to be part of such an outstanding organization. To any dentist who might be reading this book, let me tell you something. If you get involved and qualify to be part of Infinity Dental Partners, you will be happy. You do have to qualify; you're not just going to be able to come here and join the group. They're going to interview you, talk to you, and look at your financials. There is a process, but it's very fair. They want to help everyone in their organization to succeed and achieve their goals. In my case, they want to help me more than I could have ever imagined.

Jared and Elias really have a sincere attitude. Unfortunately, in today's society, you don't see that enough. We've become so skeptical as a society, that we are always asking, "What's in it for them?" or "What's their plan?" We often think, "This can't be true", "This will never happen", or "They're just lying and trying to get my money." It's unfortunate, and I'm here to tell you that you can call me up or meet with me and look me straight in the eye, and I'll tell you that I'm glad to be with Infinity Dental Partners because they're helping me make a lot of my dreams come true.

Just this week, while I'm away, we have a new associate who is coming on board. He started yesterday, and we already have six patients scheduled for him. As far as the future of my practice, I want my legacy to remain intact along with the quality of care that I provide and I know it will under the Infinity Dental Partners umbrella.

When I retire, I want my team members to stay. They will still need jobs and I want them to feel they're still cared for. I would like to stress this point to those who want to be affiliated with Infinity Dental Partners: your team members will be well treated and cared for. My team is my priority. I have been with these fine people for years, and I want to make sure they remain in good hands. I don't want their working hours and salaries cut and I don't want them to be improperly or unfairly treated.

Let's face it - somebody else taking over a practice is a major disruption. The team members typically react with, "We're going to lose our jobs and get fired. We're going to become like an Aspen Dental or some faceless corporate machine stuck in takeover mode." I know it goes through all their minds, but with Infinity Dental Partners that's just not true. Infinity is not like the typical corporate company. The difference is that Infinity Dental is run and owned by dentists. That's the big difference with Jared and Elias, and their creation. They are not a corporate entity like Aspen or Great Expressions, and all those other horrible corporate bodies.

Fears aside, what Infinity Dental say is true - your team will remain as long as they perform their jobs correctly. This is more of an integration between your practice and Infinity Dental Partners than a changeover. Everyone at Infinity Dental Partners, employees and team members, will do the right thing by your practice.

After getting involved with Infinity Dental Partners, the goal is for the dentist to eventually transition out of the practice. The dentist has to be able to learn to step back, and get less involved than usual. Your team members start to become leaders in their own right rather than the dentist being the father figure and always saying, "Come on now, you're supposed to do it this way. Did you remember to do that?"

Let me share with you an example of an occasion when I was able to step aside and let Infinity Dental Partners handle an office situation. I had a team member who really didn't want to be a team player anymore. Their Senior Facilitator was able to get actively involved. I gave my input as a way of being involved, but I was able to step back and let others handle the situation. That's the whole idea about being part of Infinity Dental Partners.

The employee ended up leaving, and we replaced her with someone who is much more of a team player.

The other good point about Infinity Dental Partners is that they have an in-depth network of people ready to help you. Jared has said to me, "You what know Tom, we're going to handle this right." They did and they handled it in a very professional way.

My point is this: you have a team behind you. There's a network of people to help you with any situation that takes place in the practice. As the senior dentist, they back you up. That's the bottom line.

You also have a network of other Infinity Dental Partner dentists. We're all part of the organization and we have the freedom to communicate with anybody in the group about any subject. You feel like you are a part of a brotherhood of dentists who are all in the same position; you can ask them detailed treatment questions and get the help you need. To be quite honest, this peer network has been quite helpful to me and I feel like I've become a better dentist because of it. We also have the Gary Kadi organization that helps us continue to grow and be pioneers in the complete health concept for our patients.

Infinity Dental Partners has changed my life and taken the pressure off of me. Now I know I'm going to be okay for the rest of my life. When I'm ready to transition out of the office, I know it will be smooth. Already, I have more time with my wife.

I feel that the price paid by Infinity for the practice was extremely fair. They're fair people. They want me to succeed and be okay. They want to help me. Nothing about Infinity Dental Partners is cut-throat. Infinity changed my life because they've lowered my anxiety levels by helping me with management. Before, as a solo dentist, I really needed to be on top of the management aspects of the practice. Needing to be on top of every single solitary thing is hard and stressful. That's no longer the case.

I like the fact that I can stay as long as I want; they won't force me out. The contract states that I can work as long as I want. I can retain my identity. They go by the philosophy that every office has its own DNA, and they don't try to change that. They don't change the name of the practice, tell you the 'new schedule', or how to practice dentistry. Patients don't have a clue that I've associated with Infinity Dental Partners unless I tell them. However, after reading this book, they will know that I'm part of a larger organization that helps me provide them with the highest quality of patient care that can be found in their community.

Dentistry is one of the great professions, but it's going to become more challenging for the individual practitioner because there are so many demands being placed on the doctor. The solo practitioner is faced with many issues: management, employees, insurance, technology, lowering overhead, etc. The cost of dental school is skyrocketing, so new dentists graduate with significant debt, which is going to make it hard for them to buy a practice. Changes in the future of dentistry will be interesting to witness. The technology of the future will be unbelievable with digital impressions, lasers, and massive computerization. It is exciting to see so much change taking place in the field of dentistry, but I believe that those dentists who are part of a great organization like Infinity Dental Partners will grow and adapt to these changes faster than the solo practitioner.

One great change already taking place is the recognition of the systemic connection between the health of one's mouth with total health. I think there will be a more integrated process between medicine and dentistry taking place in the future. When I look at the future of dentistry, I believe that it is going to be full of exciting changes, and will be an attractive field for any young person who is considering it as a career.

6

THE IMPORTANCE OF
A "SERVANT
ATTITUDE"

by Ralph D. Beadle, D.M.D.
Catlettsburg, Kentucky

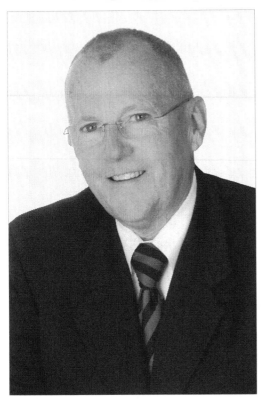

I was born and reared on a farm in the southern part of Ohio. My dad was a steelworker and a farmer; my mom was a homemaker. I was born at home with the help of our neighbor, Lizzy Walters. She was the midwife who helped bring my siblings and me into the world. I had a twin brother, but he lived for only two days. Unfortunately, healthcare wasn't at its best in those days. I had four other siblings, as well: two older sisters and two older brothers. I lost one of my older brothers when he dived from the high board into a pool, dove into a woman, and broke his neck. He was only sixteen years old at the time of his death.

My home life was very conservative, with much discipline. We had a small farm with horses, chickens, cattle, and some hogs. We went to church regularly, and I was taught to say "Yes, Sir" and "No, Sir." If I didn't speak respectfully, boy, did I get nailed! My dad worked the swing shift at the steel mill, so I would milk the cows either in the morning or in the evening, depending on his shift. When he worked the dayshift, I would milk in the morning. When he worked in the afternoon, I would milk in the evening. I got to be pretty good at it, and I made it into a game. First, I would see how much I could get into my bucket; then, I would squirt our cats and even squirt the flies on the wall. Our neighbor also had a farm, raising about 20,000 chickens, so I spent a lot of time there, as well. I like to laugh and tell people, "You know, my dad and mom only required that I work half a day, it didn't matter which 12 hours it was."

My folks were very loving, even if they were strict disciplinarians, and when I wasn't working, I liked playing sports. My dad taught me how to hunt and fish. My mom played ball, and she was pretty good at pitching horseshoes, too. I ran barefoot in the summer and I could shimmy up trees with the best of them. I guess you can say, I'm just an ole country boy.

My mom spent a lot of time with me, and she was possibly my greatest influence, especially when it came to principles and work ethic. She taught me that one's attitude is independent of the circumstances. She taught me to be reliable. I can recall many times when she would send me down to the grocery store for her and I had to be sure and give her the correct change when I returned. Whenever I was out playing with the boys in our neighborhood, I knew I had to go home as soon as I heard Mom ring the dinner bell. She taught me to have integrity, to express gratitude, to apologize when necessary, and to visualize success in life. She helped me realize that we all commit mistakes, and if we get knocked down, we get back up.

Another very influential person in my life when I was young was our pastor, Sidney Snyder, who spent a lot of time with the youth of our church. Rather than focusing on "hellfire and brimstone," he gave us very practical advice. He taught us that even when we make mistakes, it is important for us to persevere and to keep our eyes on our goal. As the saying goes, "When eating an elephant, take one bite at a time." Influences such as my mom and Sidney Snyder taught me the importance of mentors and to observe others and find out how they became successful. I learned these principles through a collection of lessons rather than one event. At the time, I didn't understand the full impact they would have on me. I do now.

I met my wife, Linda, at church when she was in fourth grade. I bought her a little box of chocolate cherries with a little stuffed dog. The cherries are long gone, but she still has that little dog. We both owned horses growing up, and on Sunday I would ride my horse over to her house and we would spend the afternoon on horseback. In September 2014, we will be celebrating our 46th wedding anniversary. Once, she asked me why I married her, and I said, "You know why! I liked you growing up, because you could run fast and you could play ball with the best of them!" Of course, back then, those things were the most important to me. I also like to tease her by telling her I had so much money invested in her that I had to marry her to get some return on my investment. Linda and I have two daughters and six grandsons, now. It's a zoo when we all get together, but they're fantastic. We also reared two foster kids: they're grown up and gone now.

As a teenager, I attended Valley High School in Lucasville, Ohio. I was the senior class president and graduated from a class of less than 100 students. (Incidentally, our 50th class reunion will be in 2014, and we are creating a book detailing the path each student has taken over the past fifty years. We have sent out questionnaires to all the students, asking about their lives, and the feedback has been very interesting.) My folks were pretty conservative in terms of Christian values, and my mother wanted me to become a minister. With this goal in mind, I went to Circleville Bible College (now called Ohio Christian University), and I completed a five-year program in four years. I soon learned that this path wasn't for me. Searching for my niche, I went to Asbury

University in Wilmore, Kentucky and earned a degree in chemistry. I was thinking about medical school at that time, and Dr. Ray, who taught biochemistry, was very influential in my life. After earning my degree in chemistry, I decided to continue on to graduate school as a doctoral candidate in biochemistry.

After three years, I realized I was tired of spending time in a lab with rats, and I wanted to be around people. At that time, my wife was a nurse who worked in oral surgery, and Dr. Ray White was the chairman where she worked. I spoke with Dr. White and he said, "Ralph, I want you to think about dental school." I hadn't seriously considered dental school before, but at that time, Kentucky offered a pace program in which a student could study at his or her own pace to acquire a degree. I had already gone through graduate school in biochemistry, so I was able to take a few exemption exams, and I graduated in three years instead of four.

When I started dental school, I was a young, married guy with a family of two little girls. Finances had to be taken into account, and at the time, the United States Army had a health profession program in which the program participant could trade each year of financial help for a year of service in the army. I was accepted into this program, and the army paid all my tuition, bought all my books, and gave me a living allowance of $460 tax-free each month. That was big money back then. Because of the military, I was able to graduate from dental school debt-free.

As I think back about why I became a dentist, I remember graduate school and my conversations with Dr. Ray White, and the soul-searching I did because I simply couldn't find my niche in life. In all of this, I realize I chose dentistry because I enjoy service, I enjoy the hands on work, and I appreciate that the financial reward is a result of the work I accomplish. In other words, it isn't simply socializing: You work and you get paid. I like that. I like the professionalism. Originally, when I was considering medical school, I realized that the lives of the medical students were completely tied down. Dentistry appealed to me because it was convenient, and I could acquire my degree earlier.

In the space of about five years, I had several major influences on my dental practice. I was able to take Zig Ziglar's "Born to Win" seminar. I also took Dale Carnegie classes and classes from Tom Hopkins and his sales techniques. One very big influence on my understanding of business was Rich DeVos and his Amway business principles. Throughout those five particular years in dental practice, I also learned the importance of a "servant attitude."

In 2007, I sold my dental practice and we left for a mission trip in Africa. During that time, my partner brought his new wife into the office, and unfortunately she and the staff had a misunderstanding and several of the staff members were terminated from employment. It was quite a blow for me, since these Team members were like family to my wife and I. They had been released without warning after having worked for me for 18 years or more. Only two weeks prior to their termination, they had been commended for the excellence of their work, and suddenly, because of unexpected drama, they were unemployed.

Several of the former Team members came to me and asked if I would open a new office. I was ready to retire at the time, but then several former patients also came to me and asked, "What happened? We need you back." I found a place that practically fell into my lap. I told the Team that I would give them five good years. They went to work and we have not looked back. It has been an awesome ride!

It was just around that time that IDP came into the picture. It seemed almost too good to be true. I will be honest, I was leery about the whole proposal, because of the recent drama in my former dental practice. I realized that I could not continue my dental practice forever. I did a lot of soul-searching, and I felt my heart was in the right place, even though I couldn't understand why. I'm a

Christian, and I firmly believe that God will unlock doors if something is meant to be. I've never received one negative experience with this belief. So, when I received a letter in the mail concerning IDP, I responded. The first person I spoke with at IDP was Randy (Jared's dad). He was relatable, positive, and personable. I was invited by IDP to send some information about myself, which I did. I was then invited to come to Michigan. When I arrived, I found everybody to be friendly and relatable. I was particularly impressed when I met and spoke with Jared (Elias was gone at the time). Every time we talked, I could see him as a partner. He even called me that. Perhaps it was a small thing to him, but it was a very big deal to me.

Never once after visiting IDP did I receive a negative vibe concerning this opportunity. The principles that the Team and IDP as a whole were promoting were exactly like mine in the realms of patient care and whole health. In the world of dentistry, we know that dental problems and dental health in general is related to the whole body. Unfortunately, this is not emphasized as much as it should be. In the big picture of personal healthcare, dentistry has a huge impact, especially when dentists themselves are up-to-date with the many issues facing the overall health of the patient. Attending a simple weekend class on these issues, I've found that I'll suddenly be faced with an issue (such as sleep apnea), and realize that dentistry can help answer the problem. In this way, if a dentist himself is up-to-date on the relationship between oral health and the patient's overall health, then the dentist can sense the needs of the patient and offer good health options. This gives me the opportunity to offer my patients various suggestions on how to improve their overall health, while at the same time respecting their right to choose what they would like to do. I never force anything on my patients. I just want to give them enough information so they can make an intelligent decision. As far as the relationship between dental health and oral health, dentists have an obligation to inform and educate patients, teaching them that what affects them orally can affect their whole body. The importance of exploring this area of health is one of the philosophies of IDP. I appreciate the help they have given me by providing materials to help patients better understand their overall health, and even the effect that dental issues can have on diseases such as diabetes, Alzheimer's, kidney disease, arthritis, cavities, head and neck pains, cancers, heart disease, etc. Education is a great part of oral health and total body wellness, and IDP has helped change the way the dental field faces these issues.

I have also appreciated IDP's philosophy on dentistry. Yes, dentistry must be viewed as a business, but it is also a ministry. My hope was to work in a place where my staff and I could have peace of mind, financially and otherwise, and IDP fit into that picture. IDP also supports the understanding that life is too short to spend it doing something you don't enjoy. This is my personal philosophy, and thankfully, IDP shares that philosophy. I'm a firm believer that there is room for improvement in every company. I have been impressed with Jared and Elias's philosophy and IDP's way of thinking. For instance, they realize that people love to get or receive little things, so we have employed a simple marketing strategy in which pens are given to patients with our name on it. This has proven to be a very rewarding marketing strategy.

When my wife, Linda, and I went to Michigan, my office manager and her husband came with me. I was open with the members of IDP, and they were open with me. I was still a little gun-shy from my experience with my last dental practice, and I kept waiting for the bomb to drop. In reality, IDP was almost too good to be true. My staff's questions were answered, and they were happy. Originally, I was concerned that I would have to let some of my staff members go. Throughout my dental practice, I have always been very open with my staff. I do not micromanage my practice. Each department is its own entity, and we are held accountable to that system. It has worked well for me over the years. For instance, if a patient disagrees with the billing, and the insurance didn't pay quite enough, then that department has the liberty to adjust the situation without running to get my permission. Then, my Team can inform me later about the situation and we can discuss it.

I always try to include the Team in decisions, hoping that they will take a sense of ownership for the work done, even though my name is on the bottom line. From the beginning of each situation, my Team knows what is going on. I ask questions, and I tell them, "Okay, this is what's happening." I always attempt to get their input. I've always used this system, and it has worked well for me. This team has taken care of me and I wanted to know that they in turn would be taken care of by IDP. Jared and Elias assured me that they would. They went so far as to say, "You've shown you had success. Let's just build on that and continue to grow and help things run even more smoothly than they are now."

Of course, it is still a new experience to be with IDP, and there are still a few mechanical bugs to work out as far as getting insurance companies to transfer checks, etc. But I have been given the liberty to handle each situation as I see fit, and that has made a difference. In one situation, our hygienist was on maternity leave and we needed to fill her position. IDP's advice was very beneficial. We ended up hiring two hygienists as the Practice has grown. The people at IDP help me to look at my options from various angles. Jared and Elias never dictate to me, and they have expressed a deep confidence in me, saying, "Hey, Ralph, you have shown us how to attain success, and you have demonstrated success. We just want to grow from that." This encouragement has made me want to succeed all the more.

Dentistry has been very good to me. I have enjoyed it immensely and I could not think of another profession where I could attain the things that I have strived to achieve. Of course, every day I try to do better and try to learn more. I had heard about a "servant attitude" before, but I didn't realize how important it could be until the past five years or so. I think it was Zig Ziglar who said, "If you give people what they want, you will get what you want." That is certainly true!

As a dentist, I have learned how important it is to have good Team members in your office: they can make or break your practice. I have learned that it is imperative to be cheerful, to maintain good eye contact, and to have a good handshake. (I am trying to teach my grandsons how important these things are. These gestures may seem small, but their impact on a person's life is not.) I have learned the importance of knowing how to relay different information to patients. Everybody wants to be healthy and to live longer. That does not simply apply to oral health. It also applies to conducting exams to detect cancer and changes in tissue. In moments like that, it is crucial to know how to relay that information to the patient. Many dentists know about the actual diseases and issues caused by dental problems, but they don't know how to relay the information to their patients. They don't always realize the need to be flexible. There are different human personalities, and these personalities must be spoken to in different ways. It is critical, when relaying information about the effects of oral health on the whole body, to be aware of the effect which word choice and voice inflection may have on the patient.

When I talk to a patient, I always put their chair higher than mine. I then sit and talk to them face-to-face. I ask them, "How can I help you?" and I listen. This has worked very well for me in building rapport and trust with my patients. I'm a firm believer that people in general, and patients in particular, don't care how much you know until they know how much you care. Of course, every professional has bad days, and I have had situations when I needed to redo crowns and dentures. I have tried to treat people the way I want to be treated, and rather than make excuses for myself when I have made a mistake, I simply accept it, redo the work, and my patients return and reward me many fold. I have learned that the important thing is to be a skilled laborer and to have good "people skills."

Unfortunately, I have noticed that some of the younger generation in dentistry seems to be concentrating more on the economic issues of the business. Of course, it's important to make a living, but that cannot be the priority. My dental practice has never suffered from any economic problems. I feel very fortunate, and I credit this phenomenon to my team for creating value for the patient. I'm a firm believer that a living is made from 9 am to 5 pm, and a fortune is made after 5 pm. I've learned how important it is to be willing to see my patients, and to be flexible. Every time I receive an emergency call, I try to work it into my schedule. Sometimes, I will stay a little longer for an X-ray and a prescription to make my patient comfortable. I will then re-schedule him or her for more permanent treatment at a later date. I've been asked to treat more crowns, more implants, etc., because I took care of my patients when they were in a time of dental crisis.

As I've said before, if you're helping enough people get what they want, you'll get the things that you want. This philosophy has worked for me and I wish I could get younger dentists to realize that. It is so simple. Take care of the patients and your Team, get the systems in place, and the stress will go down. Anytime you work with people, there is going to be some stress. Exercise people skills and flexibility and the future of dentistry is going to be there. People are going to need you. I'm speaking from the heart. These are my philosophies and my principles and they work for me. They may not work for somebody else, but I think they will.

I guess it just comes from maturing. I didn't say aging: I said maturing. (I have to chuckle as I write that.) Back when I started in dentistry, I took out teeth with no gloves on. Now, I wouldn't even think of picking up an instrument without a glove on. You need to be willing to change as paradigms change with time.

The practice was thriving, and I felt very blessed. I felt confident, invincible. Then, one evening in the autumn of 2000, I was loading some hay on the farm and I felt a pain in my jaw. The pain traveled down to my arm, and I felt sick. I was forty pounds overweight, and I knew what was happening: I was having a heart attack.

I was able to get to the house and, because we live out in the country, my wife rushed me to the hospital without waiting for the ambulance to arrive. I had some stents put in, and from that moment, my life was changed. I quickly realized, "Hey, you're not so tough and there are other people in control."

In 2006, I was having severe sinus problems and finally diagnosed as having a tumor behind the right eye. It was truly a wake-up call. The neurosurgeon was able to remove the benign, well encapsulated tumor.

These two events helped to put life in perspective. Whether it's raining or snowing, sleeting or shining, I don't care. I am just glad I'm here to experience it. I'm more relaxed. These experiences have positively affected my relationships with my patients and with my Team. These incidents have helped me to relate to my patients and to be more understanding, because, again, the patients don't care how much you know until they know how much you care.

My mother once told me, "Son, success is created by making inconvenience convenient. You have to be willing to change." As we begin our endeavors with IDP, we're still working out a few bugs in the system.. However, knowing that everybody is in the same boat and realizing that there are bumps in any road, every issue can and will be resolved. If you're flexible and have a heart that is willing to change, you will be able to easily care for your patients.

One time, I was asked how I see myself moving on. We've only been with IDP for about fourteen months now, but in the future of my practice and its relationship to IDP, I see myself improving. I have regular communications with Jared and Elias. I certainly enjoy the feedback. This feedback acts as a checks and balances. I want to make this working relationship a win-win. I don't want to simply reap all the benefits. I want to make sure that the people of IDP are comfortable and that they are receiving the benefits, as well. The patients make it a triple win.

I see a future where I can gradually phase out and be replaced by an associate. IDP has offered to find my replacement when I am ready to leave, which gives me peace of mind. As for how long I will continue in dentistry: I see myself always being welcomed in the practice. I have enjoyed dentistry and the support of IDP, and I have been relieved of many of the frustrations of the day-to-day operations of my practice by IDP. I see my patients and the Team taken care of and the practice continuing on. I certainly want to continue nurturing these relationships. With all that being said, I am unsure how long I will continue my dental practice.

In the future, I hope to take Jared and Elias to Uganda with me on a ten-day dental mission trip. It will change their lives. We're trying to establish a compound over there and I would like them to take some time to go with me. Helping others is a worthwhile experience. Of course, we'll go on some safaris, drive through Uganda, and take some boat rides with the hippos and elephants, so it won't be all work and no play. We will also have some time to, as I like to say, "Sit down and sharpen the axe."

There is a book entitled, *Don't Sweat the Small Stuff and It's All Small Stuff*. Life is too short, so let's just help people, have a good time, and make good relationships. We need to stop and smell the roses, spend time with family, and treat patients the way we want to be treated.

As I look back, I credit the events in my life with the big effect they have had on me, in my outlook, future, and my relationships with my kids, grandkids, wife, and Team. I look back and I realize that I didn't always understand what was happening at the time. Now, I see how these events have helped me relate to other people. That's how I wanted it to be, and that's how it has to be. I have peace of mind. IDP has been almost too good to be true. Over the years, I have made decisions, seen both the good and the bad aspects of these decisions, and lived with them. That is the kind of philosophy I have had, and I have certainly been blessed.

Thank you and you MAKE it a GREAT day.

7

ONE OF THIRTEEN CHILDREN

by Timothy Brunacini, D.D.S.
Hillsboro, Ohio

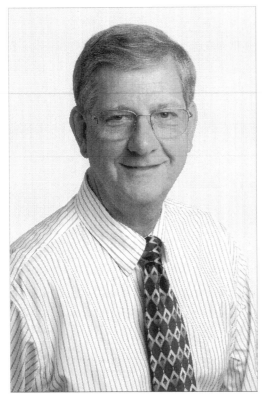

I grew up in a faith-based family in Jamestown, New York. I was the sixth of thirteen children with a stay-at-home mom and a factory dad. We would have been considered poor by today's standards, but at the time, we never felt that we were lacking anything. Growing up with such a large family was cool. We didn't have anything to compare our family situation with: None of our family members had so many kids, and some didn't have any. We were certainly celebrities: every year, when we went back to school, people would ask, "What did you have this year, another brother or another sister?" I was glad I had a lot of choices with relationships. I was, and still am closer to some siblings than others.

Growing up, there were several events that had serious impacts on me. When I was ten years old, my two-year-old sister died of Sudden Infant Death Syndrome (SIDS).

We probably had ten kids in the family at that time. Her death was a big blow, completely out of the blue, but it taught me that bad things can happen to good people. Things happen that are out of our control, and sometimes our choices in life can result in tragedies that we never anticipated.

My parents helped us to learn from this tragedy by the way they handled it. They helped us to see that we were not totally damaged. God had a reason, but since we didn't know the big picture like He did, it became an opportunity for us to grow together as a family as we dealt with the tragedy. When I look back, that was probably the biggest event in my life that changed me and made me who I am now.

When I was fifteen, my father was diagnosed with heart disease and disabled. He was forty-eight, and his diagnosis certainly made things tougher for us. My dad's early disability was another significant event in my life, because it made me realize that you're a heartbeat away from disaster. Once again, my family pulled together to face this trial. It taught me to stick with my goals, because it's important to prepare for the future.

My education from kindergarten through ninth grade involved parochial school. Each day, we would walk to church as a family, walk back home for breakfast, and then walk to school. This was our morning routine. As a teenager, I attended Jamestown High School, which was fairly large: about 650 kids per grade. The number of students helped everyone to blend in and become ordinary.

After high school, I went to community college in Jamestown for two years so that I could receive a decent education while saving money and living with my parents. My parents charged me $50 a month for rent, which I thought was awful at the time. I remember thinking "How can you charge your son $50 a month?" When I got married, they gave me all the money I had paid them for rent as my wedding gift. I thought it was a neat lesson, and it's one I will always carry with me. By charging me $50 a month for rent, they taught me the value of money and how to pull my own weight. Incidentally, I wanted to do something similar for my children, but financing our kids' education wasn't much of a factor for my wife and I. Instead, I offered my children the incentive of letting them keep 10% of whatever scholarship money they received. I figured it was a win-win: it gave our children the incentive to do well, and it helped me to offset the cost of college. My oldest son probably totaled $150,000 in scholarships, so he was able to pocket about $15,000.

I have a brother who is a registered nurse, but I was the only one out of my family to go to a four-year college, and I did it all by myself. My family wasn't able to pay for my education, though they did provide moral support throughout my school years. I was able to support myself monetarily through college, and I believe I have a more thorough appreciation for college because of the struggles I faced.

When I finished my biology degree at the University of Buffalo, I went on to dental school. In case I didn't get into dental school, I also earned a teaching certificate for secondary education: that was the best part of college for me. However, I did get into University of Buffalo Dental School, and that is where I met my partner Bob, as well as my wife.

If I had to choose the three biggest events in my adult life, I would say: Choosing to become a dentist, marrying Susan, and having children. If I had to choose a fourth event, it would be asking Bob to come and join the practice twenty-three years ago.

I've been married to Sue for thirty-seven years. We met in community college: she was in her first year, and I was in my second. I was the nerd, and she was a cheer-leader. It was one of those relationships that you never thought would happen, but did. A mutual friend set us up, and we immediately hit it off. We dated for about a year and a half, got engaged, and were married a year and a half later.

We've been together for forty-one years, and married for thirty-seven years. I'm seventy now, so this relationship has been ongoing for about two-thirds of my life. As with any marital relationship, we've had our ups and downs, but mostly ups. We've grown together, we've always been supportive of each other, and we give and take with each other. Our two children have strengthened our relationship and made things easier for us.

We're proud of our kids; they have done well. They have become successful through their own efforts. As parents, we've simply supported them, helped them realize their potential, and made them feel good about their choices. Now, they also have the support of their wives, their wives' families, and their friends. Everything has worked out well, and we feel blessed.

My eldest son is a thirty-year-old general dentist in Portland, Maine, while his wife is a public health dentist. I thought he would take over for me, but in many ways, I'm relieved that he went his own way, because his success is not tied to mine. My other son, Kevin, is twenty-seven and works in a family practice as a nurse practitioner. He is married to Andrea, who is an ICU nurse. They have been married for two years, now.

We have no grandkids yet, but we are looking forward to that. We do have two grand-dogs, though, and we spoil them like we would our grandchildren.

I chose to become a dentist because it fulfilled my need to be in the medical sciences and healing arts. It also allowed me to be more creative than I could have been in a medical discipline — which I didn't even know at the time. From the time I was in high school until I was a junior in college, I worked at a hospital, performing tasks that nowadays fall to the nurses and orderlies. I was always aware that I was intelligent enough to become a physician and I was pre-med when I thought of going out to save the world. However, by working at the hospital, I was exposed to the bad side of medicine - deaths and failures - and I didn't know if I could deal with that very well. My brother-in-law, who was eighteen years older than me, was my mentor at the time. He was a self-made man and a dentist, and he introduced me to the world of dentistry. He showed me that, as a dentist, you could be creative, healing, and provide medicine... He showed me that dentistry was a pretty good area to pursue, and my desire to become a dentist began at this time. I became committed to this idea, and when I was in my junior year in college, I chose to study dentistry.

Regarding Maslow's Hierarchy of Needs, I would say that I have attained self-actualization already. I don't have to deal with deaths, and I get to spend quality time with my family on weekends. I am able to balance work, family, and everyday living, without compromising anything. It's wonderful.

My philosophy in dentistry is simply to follow the Golden Rule. It may sound corny, but I strive to offer my patients what I would choose for myself, my wife, or my mother. I endeavor to focus on the areas of dentistry in which I excel: namely, restorative and cosmetics. In areas where I lack experience as a specialist, I prefer to refer my patients to dentists who are better informed than I am. It took some dental failures for me to realize this, but I was relieved to finally learn that I didn't have to take all of the weight on myself. The bottom line is patient care, and if another dentist can provide better patient care than I can, then I want my patients to visit that dentist.

About thirty years ago, after three years of "winging it" and trying to make dentistry work on my own, I bought into a practice in Hillsboro. The dentist who sold me the practice became my employee, and a few management programs helped to get the staff on board with the new management. The former owner retired in 1990, and I went on the lookout for a partner.

That was when I talked to Bob. He had been my friend since dental school, and we still talked to each other regularly. He had been to Hillsboro, and I had visited him. I could tell his mood had changed: he was not happy with dentistry anymore, which was unfortunate, because he was an excellent dentist.

He was living in Maryland, suburban DC, and capitation was killing him. He disliked that he was benefiting from not doing any dental work, and he felt that, as a dentist, he was almost prostituting himself. I, in turn, told him how frustrating it was to be unable to draw a quality dentist to a rural area. He commented, "I would come there in a heartbeat." I replied, "Don't say that unless you are serious, because I would love to see that happen."

I didn't think anything would come of this conversation, but he convinced his wife that it was the best thing to do. He said that coming to Hillsboro was the best thing for him and his kids. We had some reservations at the beginning; we were concerned about mixing family and business, and feared that working together would hurt our friendship. We were wrong. We have worked together for twenty-three years, without conflict, and our practice has strengthened our friendship until we've become closer than brothers. Even though my income declined with his arrival - we were splitting our gains - I would do it again in a heartbeat. This arrangement gave us the benefit of a four-days-a-week lifestyle. We were able to cover each other on vacations, and share a practice philosophy that most other dentists would envy.

In the beginning, rural dentistry occasionally had its drawbacks: It's a little harder to get labs and referrals, when you're out in the "boonies." Over the years, we've managed to establish referral patterns and overnight deliveries. The best part of rural dentistry is that you get to see the families: In our practice, we treat many families, and it is a unique privilege to see them grow and return to our practice. Our patients consist of several generations of families, right down to children who have been coming to us since they were two years old. It is wonderful to see this kind of continuity, and it's my favorite part of rural dentistry.

Within the last few years, some of our colleagues have found it difficult to find associates that see the value of rural dentistry and the lifestyle that it affords. We checked into Heartlands, Aspen, and some of the more corporate practices. The strip mall dentists were only interested in the strip mall demographics: they didn't see Hillsboro as an area that they wanted to penetrate. Then we got a cold call from Infinity Dental Partners (IDP). They were just beginning at the time, and when we didn't hear from them again for a year, we assumed they weren't interested. Frankly, no one seemed interested in us. Luckily, we found out that Infinity Dental Partners' growth necessitated a restructuring. When they were ready, they called us back, and we began communicating.

Now, I've always been more future-focused than Bob: his wife, Michelle, battled cancer for twelve years, and only recently passed away. It was difficult for him to be future-focused, when he was so enwrapped in his wife's health. Every time we had to make a decision about the future of our practice, I felt like I was grabbing him by the nose hairs and tugging him along. We would try to explore different outlets for our exit strategy, but the conversations always ended by Bob saying, "Well, let's just see what happens with Michelle." That made it kind of difficult, because we didn't have any closure or definition for our exit strategy.

Between February 2013 and now, we decided that Infinity Dental Partners provided us with an exit strategy that we liked. We liked it because we had closure, and we were given the opportunity to walk away after our two-year commitment to IDP is complete. We also have the option to continue working if we are productive and Infinity Dental Partners wants us to continue our work. We liked that freedom of choice, because neither of us can imagine hanging up the hand piece in two years. Infinity Dental Partners provided us with closure, possibilities, and also the freedom to choose to stay productive in our later years and extend our careers, if we wanted.

We had a good practice, but we knew that we had the potential for betterment and that if we kept going un-structured into our retirement years, we would probably wane rather than grow. We felt that a management company who focuses on growth would help our years to be more enjoyable, our practice to grow, and our legacy to continue. By joining with Infinity Dental Partners, our patients are cared for, and our team has options beyond our years. That is important to us and we feel that our practice can continue on even after we are gone.

Traveling to west Michigan to meet Jared and Elias (the owners of Infinity Dental Partners) was a pleasure. It was great to meet two young dentists who had their acts together; It was almost embarrassing to see where they are in relation to where I am now. The different alliances they have made are incredible, and the fact that they have accomplished so much at the young age of thirty-five is even more incredible. I was impressed with their abilities and with the way they have surrounded themselves with experts, who can provide both them and their colleagues with everything they require.

The West Michigan Summit meeting was a great experience. The meeting was an open forum, given in lecture format. Jared and Elias explained their treatment plan for a practice like ours, and gave us the chance to ask them questions. Dr. Chuck Keever was also part of this forum: he is a dentist whose practice was purchased by Jared and Elias when Dr. Keever was in his sixties. Jared had originally worked for Dr. Keever when he graduated from dental school, and now their positions have been reversed. Dr. Keever was very positive about his relationship with IDP, and said that he has seen the benefit of working for them.

Infinity Dental Partners was extremely tactful when dealing with Bob's situation with his wife's battle with cancer. I was able to relay all of the information about IDP to Bob, and when Bob was ready to move on this new idea, Infinity Dental Partners went through the information with him again. They were patient with him, helping him along and reinforcing what I had already told him. In this way, he was included in the decision-making process, rather than just accepting what I was telling him. At a time when Bob was not emotionally able to make big decisions, Infinity Dental Partners did what was necessary to make him feel comfortable.

The negotiation process started out generically - almost a template document - and the negotiations were both painless and fair to both sides. We didn't want any turmoil, and Infinity Dental Partners was very receptive of the majority of the points that we discussed.

Our greatest concerns were in regard to our staff: Most of them had been with our dental practice for thirty or forty years, and we weren't sure if they would consider this change to IDP as something that would be in their interest. We would never want to throw our staff or our patients under the bus. After meeting their senior facilitator, they seemed to join Bob and I in feeling more confident about this change. We were able to factor in everyone's needs, thus mimicking the 'four-win' mentioned in IDP's initial presentation to us: where IDP wins, patients win, the staff wins, and we win. I have great faith in this 'four-win' plan.

All of the members of IDP have been incredibly helpful and enthusiastic, and it seems that the transition of patients will be pretty seamless. By rerouting banks and routing numbers, our staff has been relieved of tasks such as month's closing and balancing budgets, leaving them time to complete other necessary tasks.

The senior facilitator who works with the practice came in and sat down with our team. He went through an overview of the processes of Infinity Dental Partners with us. Bob and I had some reservations on how the staff was going to perceive this overview, but he was able to read some of the people that were the most resistant, and at least soften them a little bit, getting them to open their minds to other possibilities. He explained the importance of working together, having common goals, and learning good communication techniques.

He re-introduced the concept of making promises and entering into agreements with each other. He suggested that we keep everything out in the open, and make agreements to do what is necessary to make sure that colleagues will not sand-bag each other's feelings down the road. IDP has offered us weekly Skype sessions, in order to follow up with us and continue our education process. That way, we can build on what we're learning, and critique our growth between meetings.

Oftentimes, the staff will think, "The doctor is excited about this idea now, but it will go away soon and things will get back to normal." Each time we have gone through a management program in the past, we have reached a plateau, and we've had to begin again from a lower level. I think there's always going to be a plateau: we can't continue infinitely. However, with IDP, I believe that our growth will continue on and we'll learn more, thanks to the follow–up meetings that will be provided. There are all kinds of positive possibilities available through IDP; I no longer dread the unknown future. I don't think the staff has enough focus on the big picture to see that yet, but I think IDP's senior facilitator has them moving in that direction. I think they will all soon see that this association with IDP will only improve their working environment.

Overall, the relationship with IDP is still playing out. I'm not sure that any real day-to-day differences have been seen yet, but I know my personal feeling of security (the warm fuzzies, if you will) has increased, and I feel that there is structure and closure coming to us in the future. That has certainly made a big difference in my well-being: now, coming into work in the morning doesn't always feel like Monday morning.

There has been some "doom and gloom" about fluorides and periodontal disease vaccines, and we may lose patients due to this negative propaganda, but I believe that, despite the propaganda, dentistry has a great future in store for it. The future of dentistry is going to be more high-tech, and more digital. More digital impressions and implants will become the standard of care. Hopefully, these improvements will bring down the price of dental care, so patients will be more receptive to these procedures and the cost will not be a barrier to patient health. Overall, I believe that dentistry has a rosy future. Otherwise, I wouldn't have suggested this career to my oldest son.

It may sound corny, but my one hope is that the Golden Rule principle doesn't change. No matter how advanced we get technologically, if we no longer have the compassion, creativity, and desire to heal and prevent disease, dentistry as a profession is not going to move forward. If we can use the technology that will facilitate important procedures, without losing sight of that principle, then I think dentistry will do fine. It will still be a good profession to pursue.

8

IV SEDATION CHANGED THE WAY I CAN HELP MY PATIENTS

by Robert G. Ross, D.D.S.

Hillsboro, Ohio

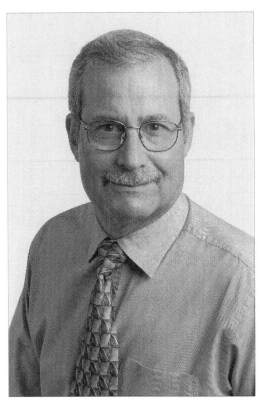

I am originally from New York, and I spent most of my childhood in the New York City area. When I was very young, my family lived in Queens; however, as the neighborhood turned "rough," my parents made the decision to move our family to Nassau County, which is one county over from Queens. It was a good place to grow up and make friends. I was your typical American kid growing up in the '50s. My mom stayed home, and she would chase me out of the house, as mothers did during the '50s, by telling me to go outside and play. I would come back with torn jeans from roughhousing and getting into minor scuffles. My father was a general dentist. He had a two-operatory practice--think of a barber-chair-type dentist office with two chairs next to each other and the dentist standing behind one of the chairs to work on a patient.

My parents were good people. They both lived through the Depression and World War II, so they had learned to live frugal lives, especially my father. Even though my father earned a good living, we were not spoiled as kids. He made sure that we learned the value of hard work and earning money. We had to work while we were in high school and in college to help pay our own way. I attended high school at Great Neck North. It was a good school, and I had many friends there. After graduating high school, I attended Lafayette College (Easton, PA) and majored in biology. It was a small liberal arts college when I was a student; however, it has grown quite a bit since then. I graduated from Lafayette in 1973 with a Bachelor's Degree in Biology. At that point, I was not sure what I wanted to do. My father was a dentist, my uncle was a dentist, and my brother was in dental school. I guess some people assumed that I would also attend dental school to follow in my father's footsteps; however, I did not want to do that at the time.

Instead, I enrolled at the University of New York in Buffalo because I was interested in biology and biochemistry. I was able to work in Roswell Park, a large cancer institute, which is similar in nature to the Sloan-Kettering or MD Anderson centers. I was in the Ph.D. program for about two years. I was still a young kid, and the long hours required for research and studies (i.e., trying to find 25 hours in a 24-hour day to work), combined with the language barrier from working with foreign physicians, began to wear on me. I began to think that research was not what I wanted to do with my life, after all.

I was living with my brother in Buffalo at that time. He was in the middle of completing his oral surgery residency, and I started getting curious about what he did. I wanted to learn more about his work. Even though I had spent a lot of time at my father's dental office, I had never known much about dentistry. Now I wanted to talk to people and learn more about dentistry to discover if this was a path that I wanted to take. It dawned on me that, as a dentist, I would have more time to spend with my family, and I would also be helping people while enjoying a productive, fulfilling career. I chose to stay in Buffalo and apply to dental school. The tuition was affordable for me, a far cry from what students are paying today, and it was a good school, so I was glad that I had made that decision.

Growing up, the greatest influences in my life were my father, and my wife. My father was very supportive and imparted many words of wisdom that I still live by today. One example in particular comes to mind. When my wife and I got married, we did not have a lot of money to pay for a wedding. Her parents did not have the funds to help very much, so we charged some of the money on a credit card. When my father found out, he went nuts. He said,

"Never do that!" He was from *that* generation--you pay your own way, and if you do not have the money for something, then you do not buy it. My father had a great respect for people, as well as a very strong work ethic. I think that influenced me as I was growing up. He was a very supportive and wonderful person, and I was proud to be his son. I lost him on July 1, the very same day that I began my residency at the hospital. He was 59 years old, the same age that my wife was when I lost her.

Equally influential in my life was my wife, Michelle. She had a great impact on my life because we met in dental school while we were still in our formative years, our mid-twenties. Sadly, Michelle was diagnosed with cancer in the year 2000 and passed away in 2013. The experience of fighting Michelle's cancer alongside her taught me patience. I had very little patience; however, when you are in the dentistry profession, you are constantly waiting on one thing or another, so developing patience is a very important attribute. The thirteen years during which Michelle battled with cancer was a difficult time in our lives, but it was also a good time, in the sense that it brought us closer together, helped us to grow, and taught us many things. Michelle and I have two lovely daughters. One lives in Chicago with her husband, a lawyer, and my first granddaughter, Hannah, who is 1 1/2 years old. My other daughter just recently moved from Cleveland to New Hampshire with her husband, an urologist who wanted to practice out East. The birth of our daughters was probably the other event in my lifetime that had a profound effect on me. It is wonderful to see how our daughters have grown up through their immature, troublesome teenage years to become well-adjusted, responsible, happy adults. I like to think that Michelle and I imparted some wisdom that helped them as they were growing up, just as my parents did for me. In the part of rural Ohio where we lived, we saw a lot of kids who unfortunately followed the wrong path. I think that the positive way in which our daughters turned out speaks to how well we raised them. I am proud to be their father.

I had several jobs before finally opening my own dental practice. My wife wanted to live closer to her family, so we moved to Maryland. As a resident, I moonlighted at a drug store in Bowie, Maryland. It was an odd place, somewhere between a Sears and a drug store that had a small dental clinic. I would finish my residency during the day before going to work at the clinic from 7 PM to midnight. After I completed dental school and my residency, I took several different jobs as I tried to get my feet wet and decide exactly what I wanted to do as a dentist. I worked for three other dentists who needed associates. For three years, I also worked for the Department of Corrections in Maryland as a part-time dentist in a maximum-security prison in Hagerstown,

Maryland. My time at the prison, working with inmates, was definitely an eye-opening experience for me.

Unfortunately, I was driving constantly between jobs, and that kept me from seeing my family and spending much time with my girls when they were very young. That is when I came to realize that I did not want to work for other people; I wanted to be my own boss. Therefore, I opened up an office in Frederick, Maryland. At that time, Frederick was a small town with only six dentists serving the entire community. Once I had made that decision, I cut back on my associate jobs and opened the doors of my practice without even a single patient. I did keep my job with the prison for a while in order to maintain a guaranteed income for my family while I was growing my own practice. After ten years of working out of my office in Frederick, I sold my practice to my associate and moved to Ohio with my wife so that she could complete her Doctoral Degree in Education Administration. Until we moved, my wife was driving daily to the Pentagon area of D.C., and I was traveling north about 40 miles to Frederick, so we rarely saw each other. The move to Hillsboro, Ohio, would mean that she could finish her degree and that our family would all be in one place. Of course, we left Maryland with two screaming elementary-school girls who did not want to leave their friends for a strange home and a new school.

In hindsight, this was probably one of the best decisions my wife and I ever made for our family. Tim Brunacini, a friend from dental school, needed someone to work in his practice with him; my wife wanted to finish her degree; we wanted to spend more time together as a family; and my associate wanted to purchase my practice. All of the pieces fell into place so smoothly that we were left with no choice but to follow them to our new home. Our girls flourished in Ohio. People in D.C. and suburban Maryland are extremely competitive, and such an environment is not always good for raising a family. In Ohio, our daughters easily made friends (to this day, they are still in contact with many of their friends from high school), and I was able to leave behind the high-pressure competitive area for something that I much preferred: rural and semi-rural dentistry. I worked with Tim to grow our practice, while Michelle completed her Doctorate and took a job as a school administrator, in which capacity she worked until her passing about 15 years later. I have remained here in Ohio for 23 years, continuing to practice dentistry in the area that I grew to love.

I have very seldom strayed from my philosophy of dentistry. I think of my patients as if they were my mother, my brother, my family members, and I ask myself, "How would I treat you if you were my family?" I once overheard one of my assistants, who has been with us for 12 years, explaining to a patient that, "Dr.

Ross is going to talk to you just like you are related to him." I feel good about that because it makes me realize that I am giving my best to my patients. One of the biggest complaints that I hear from patients in general is that no one takes the time to explain things to them. Much to the contrary, my staff is often buzzing me, saying, "Get going, Dr. Ross; you are behind again!" I may talk too much for some people, but I know I am just taking the time necessary to make sure my patients understand and feel secure. I also try to think of the care I give to my patients and the treatments that I recommend outside of the economic aspect of the practice. I am not a specialist in all areas of dentistry, so I try to give my patients all of the options that I can and to let them know what I can accomplish for them versus what they may need a specialist to do.

Dental school teaches only one thing--treat the patient. In a perfect world, that would be an ideal way to practice dentistry. Unfortunately, some patients are unable to afford the treatment that they need because they are financially strapped. In cases like this, I give them recommendations for less expensive options that can be done before moving to the ideal plan later on. However, I never perform procedures that patients demand if I feel the treatment is not the best way to go, such as removing all of a patient's teeth just because he wants his teeth out!

I explain to my patients that I have to sleep at night and look at myself in the mirror each morning!

One thing I found that I could not accomplish for all of my patients was to reduce their anxiety about having dental treatments. I tried taking oral sedation courses and other courses along those lines and found them to be only semi-effective. They worked all right for some patients, while for others, they did not work at all. I then decided to be trained to administer IV sedation. That one simple decision has made a real difference in my ability to help my patients achieve needed treatments. Some of my patients need IV sedation due to anxiety. Over the course of employing this method, I have seen several patients graduate from needing to be sedated to needing nothing but local anesthetics. I think it is a simple matter of building trust with your patient. When they realize that their treatment went fine while they were sedated, they become confident enough to try a local anesthetic the next time around. Many of the fears that patients have of dental work comes from a bad past experience with another dentist. Once my patients learn to trust me, they see that they do not need IV sedation. However, having IV sedation available does have a definite impact on my practice.

Approximately 50% of people do not go the dentist. Some may not have dental insurance or the money to pay for dental care, but I believe that this is mostly due to fear and anxiety. Having IV sedation means that I can treat more patients by providing them with valuable much-needed, services. Another way I use IV sedation is to help patients who have schedules that do not permit them to make repeated visits to the dentist office for treatments. There are many patients who need several dental treatments that would be impossible to do in one sitting because the strain of keeping their mouths open that long would be physically impossible, or at least extremely uncomfortable. By and large, the biggest percentage of patients that are sedated do so because of anxiety; however, I also leave this option open for patients who want to have multiple treatments done in one afternoon–for example, the businessman who works in Cincinnati every day and needs several dental treatments. We can either schedule him for several repeated visits to the office, or we can sedate him and perform all of the necessary work in just 3 to 4 hours. This helps greatly when people cannot afford to take time off work or out of their schedules for repeated trips to the dentist office for treatments.

I wish I had made the decision to become trained in IV sedation earlier in my career. I am not sure where some patients get the idea that dentists stand on their chests while the patient clutches the chair, but some of them have that idea so embedded in their heads that sedation is the only way they can receive the dental treatments they need. IV sedation has made a big difference in my practice by helping me understand what my patients need.

As with any job, I guess that after a while, you become set in your ways and even experience stages of burnout. Yes, this happens even to dentists! However, when I added sedation to my practice, it helped me emotionally. I enjoy working now more than ever before because IV sedation has helped me realize more about what my patients need, whether they are sedated or not. It was a good choice both for me and for those whom I treat.

As a matter of fact, out of 10,000 dentists in Ohio, only about 300 provide IV conscious sedation. The closest dentist to our practice that provides this service is in Cincinnati, which is an hour away. We provide a service for people in our semi-rural area that they would not otherwise be able to achieve without driving over an hour away from home. There are several dentists I know that perform oral sedation; however, I believe that is too risky because you do not have the same type of control that you do with IV sedation.

As you can tell, I value my patients, and their on-going care was a major concern for both my partner Tim and for me. In terms of retirement, you worry about how your patients will be treated by a new dentist and how you will take care of your practice if you are no longer there to supervise the day-to-day operations. You worry about finding the right person to take over your practice, someone whom you can trust to treat your patients as you have treated them for many years. Your practice is like your child, in a way, and you want to make sure that it will be in good hands when you leave. Tim and I were also concerned about our staff – we had worked with these people for most of our lives, and we wanted them to continue to have jobs that they enjoyed for as long as they wanted to work.

Therefore, Tim and I started evaluating possible exit strategies. We considered taking our practice to the corporate level; however, we were concerned that our practice would not be what we had created and worked for many years to build. Then we came across Infinity Dental Partners and ended up affiliating ourselves with their organization. Infinity Dental Partners put our minds at ease regarding all of the retirement concerns we'd been entertaining.

Although we have only recently become affiliated with Infinity Dental Partners, I believe that Infinity Dental Partner's intent is to allow us to continue to practice the way we were before the acquisition. Our patients are treated the same way, and the legacy of our practice will still be what we created it to be. This is definitely not the impersonal corporate relationship that I have heard of in the past. It is not a storefront in a strip-mall-type of entity. I have patients who have been treated at dentist offices like that, and they complain that they never see the same dentist twice. There is usually no continuity of care in offices like that, so the patients end up coming back to our office. I believe that in those practices, there is also a tendency to up-charge procedures and to view the patient as a warm body instead of a real person. Those practices try to move forward with treatments regardless of what the patient may really need. I am not implying that all corporate practices are this way, but, from what I have seen, this has been my experience. However, I believe Infinity Dental Partners is very different. I feel as if I am being treated as an individual when I deal with the staff and individuals from Infinity Dental Partners. I am not talking to a corporate manager who is not a dentist and does not understand what I am dealing with in my practice. It is reassuring to know that I can work as long as I want to work and then slow down when I feel it is time, knowing that my practice will continue along in the same vein that I have worked hard to achieve for it.

Another of my concerns was my staff. You cannot be a dentist and practice by yourself. You must have a good support team, and my staff has been great. They are a part of the reason that I have a successful dental practice and that our patients are satisfied with our services. I appreciate that Infinity Dental Partners has supported me in this concern, as well. Infinity Dental Partner's support team in Michigan has been great and has answered all of my questions and addressed my concerns during the transition. That has been a very positive aspect of the transition. Our relationship with Infinity Dental Partners has been very good so far, and I expect that to continue into the future.

When we were considering Infinity Dental Partners, the phrase they used was "We're not going to change the genetics of your practice or the relationships you created." A fear that I believe many dentists have when considering transitioning into a corporation is that their practices will change and that the corporation will try to tell the dentists exactly what must be done and how to practice. Our practice, on the other hand, was based on close-knit relationships within the community, which is important to me because I do not feel you can practice without the support of your community, especially in a small environment like ours. Infinity Dental Partners has supported me in that, as well, and I am extremely appreciative. At one time, we were considering another corporation; however, they wanted to make many changes in our practice, and that did not feel right. Infinity Dental Partners understands that they must treat each practice, each dentist, as an individual. You cannot rubber-stamp directives for all practices to follow because a practice here in Hillsboro, Ohio, is much different from a practice in

New York State or in Alabama. There must be some type of leeway to allow for the differences that are inherent in each dental practice. I think Infinity Dental Partners has accomplished that very well at the corporate level.

Frankly, I do not think that any other corporation has been able to accomplish this concept the way Infinity Dental Partners has. There was a very good PBS broadcast about corporate dentistry that aired about a year ago. It was very uncomfortable to watch because it painted an extremely unfavorable picture of corporations in the dental practice, which led to some corporations being banned from practicing dentistry in several states due to the abuse of dental patients. Infinity Dental Partners is a very different environment from the one portrayed in the PBS program. From what I have witnessed so far, Infinity Dental Partners knows the health practices that they operate and how each practice treats their patients so that they can be assured that their practices are providing quality dental services.

During my 34 years of practice, I have seen many changes in the dental field and the health field in general. One of the major changes has been due to governmental medical programs and health insurance companies. Because of Medicare, Medicaid, HMOs, and PPOs, the medical industry has had to deal with mandates and changes that they may not necessarily see as beneficial to their patients.

Fortunately, dentistry is still, in most cases, an elective treatment. While some people will have emergencies that must be treated, for the most part, patients choose whether or not to see a dentist. Therefore, these changes in insurance have affected the practice of dentistry far less than the medical profession in general. Our practice has had to make some adjustments--you do that for your patients when you are in a community, and most people in that community have the same insurance company--but overall, we have had far fewer disruptions to our services when compared to other medical providers. We find that if a patient wants a certain treatment, he or she will typically find a way to pay for that treatment.

I would still advise students who are interested in dentistry to proceed with their education and enter the dentistry field. Many people have feared that the government and insurance companies would change the way dentists practice. Although this has been the case, to some degree, the dental field has not been affected like many other medical fields. I believe this trend will continue into the future, making dentistry a very good profession to enter. However, I do believe what will change going forward will be the way dentists enter private practice. The way I see it, corporate entities such as Infinity Dental Partners, will become the norm rather than dentists who hang up their shingles the way I did 34 years ago. I believe that dentistry has a very good future. I think that the more dental health is correlated to overall health, the greater the incentive will be for people to seek regular dental checkups and care. The media is currently helping us out by promoting dental care as necessary for overall health.

Your mouth is part of your body, and what happens in your mouth affects your entire body. For example, a patient may have an oral infection that results in hospitalization and surgery in order to treat the problem. I think this is a harsh way for individuals to realize that they should take care of their mouths as part of their overall health routines. I think that the dental field has recognized this change, as well. This concept makes sense to me because you are taking dentistry beyond the mouth and training doctors to look at a patient's overall health rather than simply his or her teeth. I think this is a positive change in the dental field and one that must be embraced by dentists. Dentists need to be more aware of their patients' medical situations in order to treat them accordingly and in the best way possible.

I want to leave you with an amusing, albeit chilling, memory from the time I spent working as a dentist at the maximum-security prison. I had never been inside of a jail, much less a prison. They offered me the job, and I thought "Oh, well, it is dentistry," so I accepted. I actually learned a lot while I was working at the prison. I probably extracted five thousand teeth during my few years there. In dental school, I only extracted about five teeth total, so the prison was a great training ground for me. On my first day, I arrived to meet the warden; he was a former Marine Sergeant, so you can imagine his personality. You probably need to have that type of background to be in charge of a locked down, maximum-security prison. The medical unit had 20 hospital beds and a dental clinic. In addition to me, the prison employed a few nurses and a physician. Of course, I am a dentist, so I showed up in a shirt and tie just as I would in a private practice. The warden walked over to me and said, "You need to change that," making reference to my attire. When I asked him why, he grabbed my tie, yanked on it and replied, "Because you'll get choked to death, that's why."

In that moment, I transformed from a naïve, post-dental graduate to a dentist in the real world. During residency, you see patients, but you really do not see the real world. In practice, you begin to see the real world, but because of my time in the prison, I was thrown into the real world a bit faster than would have been the case had I begun in a private practice. However, it was a very interesting time for me; I met some truly bizarre people, but yet I learned a lot about dentistry. It was an experience that shaped me and set the stage for my career as a dentist.

9

HOMETOWN BOY RETURNS HOME TO PRACTICE COMPLETE HEALTH DENTISTRY

by Grant K. Gillish, D.D.S.
Whitehall, Michigan

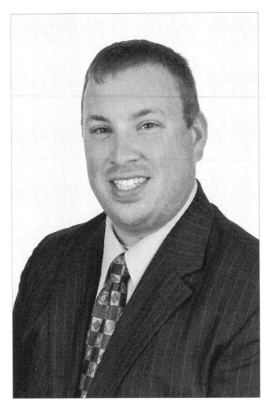

During the first several years of my life, I lived with my mother and father in Mona Shores, MI. Then, when I was in the first grade, my father's career made it necessary for my family and me to move to New York. I lived in New York for a couple of years—not in the city, but way out in the country. I have two younger brothers, and I had normal brother experiences with them: roughhousing, playing outside, and not always getting along. They are probably the two adults who, aside from my wife, I feel closest to today. I'm really happy to have grown up with them, and to have shared all the different experiences of childhood and adult life with them.

We moved back to Michigan after only a year or two in New York. This time, my mom, brothers, and I lived in Montague, Michigan—the hometown of both my parents, as well as my father's parents. I have a long history in

Montague, and the majority of my school experience took place there. I went to Montague Elementary School, starting in third grade, and I attended Montague High School. Throughout high school, I had a lot of friends, played football, fished, boated, spent a lot of time at the beach, and basically did everything that normal small town kids do. I don't think I was sheltered; I just didn't have a very broad view of life outside of a small town. When I was a junior in high school, I took my ACT and began preparing for college.

In general, I didn't feel challenged in high school, and I knew that I wanted to have a career that would be exciting and challenging, requiring a higher education and a little more thought than many of the blue-collar factory jobs that were available. I didn't want to do the same thing every day, so I considered going to medical school, law school, and possibly even pursuing a PhD in one of the sciences and becoming a researcher. As I began looking into these fields, I spoke with our family physician and with some other doctors and lawyers that my family knew. It seemed like these professionals were working long days and even weekends; they were always on call and always needed at the hospital. After talking to them, I realized that, although their careers seemed challenging and rewarding, the common thread was that their families suffered for their careers.

My mother had a very good friend from high school whose husband was a dentist. He was a really nice guy, was well respected in the community, and had a great sense of humor. To my eyes, he seemed to be a hard worker who really enjoyed his job, but at the same time, he was still able to have a family and to spend time with them. He had all the "toys" that I thought were cool and fun at the time, and we used to snowmobile with him. He had a life outside of his career, and I was really inspired by that. I realized that, unlike the other professional careers I was looking into, dentists didn't have to sacrifice their families or their lives outside of work. This appealed to me because family was so important to me. For these reasons, I decided to become a dentist, and once I made that decision, I went full steam ahead to make it happen.

I graduated high school in 2004, and was accepted to the University of Detroit Mercy. There, I received my undergraduate degree, as well as my dental school education. The university has a unique dental program. It has a six-year doctoral bachelor program, to which you can apply after you have been accepted to the regular undergraduate school. When I applied for the undergraduate program, I also applied for the six-year program. Once I was accepted into the undergraduate program, I started the interview process to be accepted to the six-year program.

First, a candidate for the six-year program has an interview with a science professor at the undergraduate college. Mine happened to be with my organic chemistry professor, which was good, because organic chemistry is one of the more challenging prerequisites for dental school. I also had an interview with a professor at the dental school. This all took place while I was still in high school. Both professors recommended that I be accepted to the six-year dental program, and I was later selected by the committee to be part of that program.

There were 107 applicants for the six-year dental program, and six of us were initially accepted. Through attrition and transferring, only four of us actually made the transfer from undergraduate studies to dental school. So out of 107 people who wanted to be part of the program, only four of us graduated from dental school in the sixth year. In this program, the undergraduate studies are a bit more challenging: the student still has to complete all of the required prerequisites for dental school. Thankfully, there is no need to attend the full four years to gain a bachelor's degree. As long as the prerequisites are complete and the student has an acceptable score on the DAT, a spot in the dental school is guaranteed. If any of those requirements is not met, then that spot is taken away and made available to someone who is on the waiting list.

Graduating from high school, I had a place reserved for me in the dental school class of 2010: I just had to meet all the requirements of my undergraduate studies. I began studying at the University of Detroit Mercy in the fall of 2004, and I had completed all of my undergraduate studies by the spring of 2006. That meant I had to take a pretty heavy course load in the fall and winter semesters, and I took classes all summer long as well. It was a bit more demanding than most undergraduate course work, but I felt it was worth it. It allowed me to be out in the workforce, practicing dentistry two years earlier than most people in dental school.

Growing up primarily in a single-parent home with my mother, I saw how hard she had to work to provide the things that we needed. The way that my mother provided for me really instilled a sense of work ethic and pride in me, as well as the desire to provide for my own family as an adult. It inspired me to show the same kind of compassion and care for my family that she showed to me.

I also wanted to help people, because, growing up, we didn't always have the best insurance or medical coverage or a ton of money to spare. I thought that, if I were in a position to help people in the way that I am now able to — providing dental care for underprivileged children and families — it would allow me to make an impact on other people's lives, the way that my mom and our family made an impact on me.

One particular event really put things in perspective for me. I had a very close friend in college who moved away for a job. We still kept in touch but didn't see each other very often, and not long after he moved away, he committed suicide. He was a really close friend—we always picked on each other and poked fun at each other—but I never really had a chance to tell him how important his friendship and our time together was to me.

Since then, I've tried to avoid taking for granted the friends I have and the time I spend with them, as well as the interactions I have with people whom I might unknowingly influence. It has made me more grateful for what I have and for the happiness that I find with the people who are important to me. His death was the first time in my life that I realized that everything that we do and everything that we are, now and in the future, has a profound effect on others, and it really made me reassess my own relationships.

Now, I try to be a little more open with people about how I feel about them and how important they are to me, because everyone needs to hear that. I don't think that I had any effect on my friend in the decision he made, but I think that maybe just being a little bit more open, honest, and caring with people is extremely important in this day and age. I think this is especially true because of how differently we interact with one another today through social media, communicating in ways that don't involve face-to-face contact. Human interaction is really important, and I've been trying to instill this realization in my own life while also communicating it to other people.

One of the major turning points in my adult life has been my marriage. Cassie is a huge part of my life. We started dating when we were in high school, and unlike most couples, we weren't on and off in our relationship: we stayed together all through college, and when we graduated, we moved back home and got married. We had been dating for about six years when I decided to propose to her. I bought a ring in June and I planned a little four-day weekend trip to Traverse City, Michigan, with the ruse of going up there for a wine tasting. When we finally went in August, we booked a nice hotel room (a little nicer than I would spring for normally), went out to dinner, and then went up to the lighthouse at the end of Old Mission Peninsula in Traverse City.

We walked about a hundred yards up the point and onto the bay in Lake Michigan. I had brought a disposable camera with me, and I asked Cassie to stand on a large rock that was in knee-deep water, so I could take her picture. She was completely confused as to why I would want to get a shot of her on that rock. The sun was just going down, so I told her to turn around and I'd take a picture of her looking at the sunset. When she turned back around, I had taken the ring out of my pocket. I proposed to her and of course, she said yes. That was the beginning of the second half of our weekend in Traverse City, which we celebrated as a newly-engaged couple.

We were engaged for about two years and got married on October 2, 2010 in the church that her grandparents had co-founded. We had the reception at the Grand Haven Community Center with all of our friends and family. It was an awesome celebration: we were so happy, and we got to share it with all the people who are closest to us.

Now, we live in Spring Lake, Michigan, with our two dogs. We don't have children yet, but we would like to have a family someday. We still spend time with both of our families, and right now our two most important little monsters are my sister-in-law's children, our five-year-old nephew and our three-year-old niece. Now that Cassie and I are married and living together, we're starting our own life: even spending time together and holiday traditions are changing, as we learn to become a family, rather than just being someone's significant other.

During my last semester at UDM, like everyone else, I started to look for work after graduation. I had an interview with one of the big chain dental companies that operate throughout the country, and I was actually offered a job in two different places. My wife and I toured the towns where the jobs were located, and were starting to consider one of these towns as a place to live when I got a phone call from Dr. Elias Achey.

It turned out that one of my grandfather's good friends, somebody whom I had gone on fishing trips with and had known for a long time, was a patient at an Infinity Dental Partners Office—the office where I currently work, White Lake Family Dentistry. He joked with Dr. Achey, saying, "Hey, how come it took me two months to get in to see you? You are so busy, you can't even be bothered to see one of your favorite patients?"

Dr. Achey responded, "Well, I'm really swamped and we are booked out a long time and there's more work than I think I can handle on my own." Just jokingly, he said, "Do you know anybody who is a dentist and is looking for a job?"

It so happened that this gentleman called my father, got my phone number, and gave it to Dr. Achey. It's crazy, these small town connections! Dr. Achey asked a few more patients from the area about me: who I was, what I was about, and the kind of person that I was. I assume he received positive reviews, because he gave me a call while

I was visiting home (I was still in dental school at that time). He and I talked for a while on the phone, and we decided that he and his wife would meet Cassie and me at a restaurant for dinner.

There was a stark difference between my interviews with the big dental chain and with this informal get-together for a meal, a few drinks, and a conversation with another dentist and his wife. This wasn't a big corporate entity that sent a human resources person to interview me: It really struck me that he was working in my hometown, that he had asked about me, and that he knew of me. I was talking to a real dentist, who interacted with his patients, knew who they were, and knew who I was. That small town, homey feel was really important to me. I felt that I could fit in really well with this company. I turned down my job offer with the nationwide dentistry chain and accepted a job with Infinity Dental Partners. This company took me under its wing and taught me a lot, giving me every opportunity to succeed, and providing complete autonomy over my treatment plans. I could provide patient dental care the way I wanted to do it. I was able to use the materials and techniques that I was comfortable with and utilize what I had learned in school. In addition to that, I was also encouraged to try new techniques, new materials, and new ways of doing things.

Infinity Dental Partners is a group of dentists who unselfishly share their knowledge and give their time to help one another become the best dentists they can be. I'll give you one example. Dr. Chuck Keever is a dentist at Infinity Dental Partners who has been practicing for a long time in Muskegon, which is only thirty minutes away from where I currently practice. He's a Las Vegas Institute (LVI) graduate dentist and he has an immense amount of knowledge and experience. The opportunity for me to ask him questions, to learn from him, and have him show me different techniques, different tools, and different ways of doing things is amazing. Dr. Keever and I get together for special cases on our days off, in order to help me to broaden my experience. I don't believe that many dentists have that opportunity.

As a dentist, if you hope to own or purchase a single-dentist practice from the current owner, you will not receive this same level of support. The nice thing about Infinity is that there is more than one person to help you: you can learn from everyone. At Infinity Dental Partners, there are dentists whose primary practice is really difficult prosthetic cases, dentists who specialize in TMJ, and dentists who are really good with kids. There is such a variety of people to learn from and bounce ideas off that it's like having your own private network of dentists who each has his or her own individual mini-specialty. It has really helped me to broaden my own experiences, and learn more than I could have in any other organization. It's an experience that I don't think anyone can have by receiving insights and tips from only one dentist.

On the other hand, the dentists in dental chains are treated simply as employees. They are told when to work and they have to apply for time off. At Infinity Dental Partners, I set my own schedule. I can take time off whenever I want. I have the autonomy to work the way I want to work on the days that I'd like to work, and there is no strong-arm human resources department telling me what I can and can't do. Some of the folks that I graduated with work for the large national chains, and they don't even work with an older dentist. Their knowledge is limited to what is available at the office and to the continuing education classes and seminars they attend. It is the only advancement that they are able to seek out. I feel it's important to stay current through continuing education, and going beyond the minimal requirements. I think it's vital to continue to improve, both as a dentist and in my personal life: I never want to be stagnant. In dentistry, there is no reason for anyone to ever be bored. There are always new technology advances available, and different perspectives to explore. At Infinity Dental Partners, I am given the freedom to follow the career path I want to follow, but with the comfort of the huge safety net of an entire community of experienced dentists.

Dentistry is an exciting field. We're on the leading edge of technology, scientific research, and material manipulation, and I'm happy, proud, and excited to be part of an industry that isn't afraid of change, and that embraces new techniques, new technology, and fresh ideas. I think that in a world that is constantly changing and altering in the areas of business, available materials, and communication, we must also continue to change and alter. It's the only way to meet the demands and the changing needs of society and healthcare as a whole.

I have several friends from my dental school, but one in particular with whom I still keep in touch on a regular basis. He was hired by a community clinic in another state, and recently, we called each other and shared our work experiences. It was like night and day. His work consists mostly of old-school amalgams and extracting teeth. In my first year, the Infinity Dental Partners sent me to a variety of continuing education courses. I learned a lot of new things like the CAD/CAM dentistry, the CEREC machine, implants, and so on. My classmate had the same education I did, graduated at the same time, and started working at the same time; and yet, because of Infinity Dental Partners, I am years ahead of him from the dental standpoint, based on the amount and variety of experiences I have had. I have been using brand new, top-of-the-line technology, and he has been using techniques that are as old, if not older, than some of the techniques that we were told were outdated when we were in dental school.

There are a wide variety of practices across the country, and I feel that Infinity Dental Partners is right at the top, at the height of technology and information. Folks that are working in the large clinics run by national chains seem to be hindered by the bureaucracy and the necessities of the business model. There seems to be no place for a dentist to have the opportunity to work in his or her own way, while also having the support of a large group of experienced and knowledgeable independent dentists, as we have with Infinity Dental Partners.

We can provide top quality, technologically advanced care. People love to play with gadgets—iPhones, iPads, tablets, and computers. Gadgetry is one of the biggest ways that people spend their time and money. New technology is one way to keep people interested in dentistry: not only dental professionals, hygienists, assistants, and people in the industry, but also our patients. Many people find the dental necessities of different lasers, digital x-rays, intraoral cameras, spectra, and 3D-imaging, very exciting.

There has never been a time in human history where information is more freely and readily available. You can learn anything you want online, and most people with smartphones and tablets have the ability to find that information instantaneously. Most people, including me, rarely go to a place of business or a restaurant without having looked it up online, found reviews, and gotten some information prior to entering the establishment. This same tactic applies to dentistry. As a dentist, imagine what happens when you recommend a treatment and then step out of the room. In the short period of time between when you leave the room and when you return, most people have accessed unlimited information about your suggestion. They have found different kinds of treatments, information about treatments, and alternatives to the treatment you suggested—even reviews, and horror stories. As dentists, it's important for us to provide as much education and information as possible to our patients, so they don't accept as gospel all the misinformation that is out there.

It's also important to manage the information online. The better the level of care you provide and the happier everyone is with you, the more the positive reviews are going to show up. It only takes one negative review to turn someone away. If people see a lot of glowing, positive comments about your practice, you are more likely to get new patients who are doing their research and are shopping around for a dentist.

I feel that there are a lot of different things that dentists can provide that are not just the nuts and bolts of dental care. One very important aspect of the dental practice is personalized care. We provide a sense of security for people. A lot of folks are very afraid of dentists and dentistry. It's important to have a close-knit dental family where patients feel comfortable and secure. Otherwise, some folks might go long periods of time without seeking care. Working in the same town that I grew up in, I see people that I went to high school with, my friends' parents, and even people that I worked with in former jobs: at the hardware store, on the celery fields, or in the asparagus field. They love to come to me and see me for their care because I understand them. I know them. We grew up in the same area, know all the same people, have some of the same experiences, and maybe even have a similar view of the world. I feel that a personal connection with people—not just the professional connection—is something that dentists should have.

Even though many dentists do develop personal relationships with their patients, having those personal relationships prior to becoming a dentist has been very beneficial for me. It has a big impact on the way I work and the way I interact with my patients. Every dentist should strive to provide personalized care. It's easy to look at a mouth and know what's wrong and fix the problems, but it's more difficult to manage a patient as a whole—as a specific person, with general health, hobbies, habits, and personalized needs. As a profession, we need to broaden our treatment plan. A lot of people talk about smoking cessation or dietary nutritional counseling. These, along with other issues, need to be implemented into our treatment plans, to make our patients feel that we care about them and want to help them to be more proactive in their own health. In general, we need to influence our patients on their entire health and total body wellness.

It seems like dental care is becoming less of a reactive treatment option and more proactive. We see more people taking care of issues early, before the issues become real problems. The public is becoming more aware of the systemic link between dental diseases and other disease in the body. It's important that we're able to promote not only oral health but also total body health. We're moving away from simply fixing and pulling teeth, and moving deeper into preventive care and total health and wellness. I think it's a good change and I look forward to continuing in that direction.

As dentists, it's also important to give back to our communities and provide access to dental care for people who can't afford it. Free dental day is an event held annually by Infinity Dental Partners. On that day, the dentists of our company join together and open the office on a Saturday. We provide dental care, free of charge, to patients in our community and the surrounding communities. We advertise a couple of months in advance and we try to see as many people as we possibly can.

It's a really hectic, long day, but it's also very rewarding. For the last few years, we've had general dentists volunteer their time and we've also had an oral surgeon volunteer his time. This year, we are doubling the size of our free dental day so we can provide even more care for more patients. It's primarily for patients with low to no incomes, and poor to no dental insurance. Our goal is to care for those people in our community who, otherwise, would not get any dental care.

In the past, we have had people travel as long as four hours because a family member in our area told them about our free dental day. All of these patients were very much in need and were so grateful for the care we provided. They also helped us get positive feedback about our office and gave us the kind of gratitude that you would never think to expect. It was amazing to see how thankful people are when they are provided with something that they really can't do for themselves. It's such an awesome experience and I'm excited to do it again this year. I believe that more dentists in the country should be a little more giving, and a little more conscious of the needs in their own areas.

Working for Infinity Dental Partners has been a wonderful opportunity for me, and I have been nothing but pleased with the way the dentists of this company operate. All the dentists in this network have allowed me to broaden my horizons from a dental and personal standpoint. The sheer magnitude of knowledge and experience that the doctors at Infinity Dental Partners have is incredible. They have provided me with a wealth of information, ideas, and input on treatments, treatment plans, and patients. It is a huge support net under me. I have the abundant experience and the different backgrounds of all the doctors at my fingertips, and can receive invaluable information and support from them. I've met a lot of really good and knowledgeable people, and I feel like I'm part of something that's important; I'm part of something that's helping my community. I am helping to provide necessary services and promote overall health and wellness, not only in my community, but also all over the country. It's an awesome experience.

Obviously, everyone is a little bit different. But personally, I would say this: If you are an individual who wants to have autonomy, and who wants to practice in a place where you're not just a producer for a large company, then you should become associated with Infinity Dental Partners. They want you to care about your patients, and provide the best quality service and care. It's an organization where you have the ability to learn from and share ideas with experienced dentists, who perhaps work in a different demographic or different area than you. There is so much you can do: work as hard as you want, do as well as you can, and really be your own person, while still being a part of something that's bigger than you are. If dentists want to continue to be where we are now— representing the top level of health care and the only refuge for people in need of oral care—we need to adapt, evolve, and increase our access and availability. And I think that's where we're headed.

10

PEANUT BUTTER AND JELLY SANDWICHES

by Neeta Chesla, D.D.S.
Spring Lake, Michigan

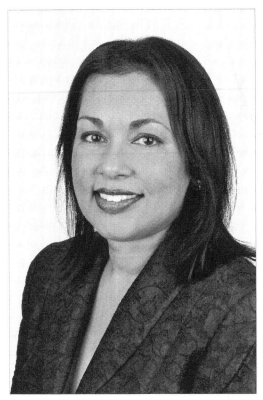

T he course of my life has changed drastically over the years. I was born in India, where my father worked as an accomplished chemical engineer. By the time I was 9, he was recruited to work in the United States and we moved to Detroit, Michigan. Our life in Michigan was very different from our life back home. In my native country, we had a nanny who took on most of the housework while I focused on playtime, school, and family. With no nanny in Detroit, we had to adjust and learn how to wash dishes, do chores, and clean our home.

Since we were privileged in India, I had a tutor before turning three. Beyond that, I attended private school. I began the fourth grade in India and had a long vacation before traveling to the United States. Once in Detroit, my parents convinced the principal at my new school to start me in the sixth grade.

On my first day of class, I remember Mr. Mastering introducing me to the students. When he mentioned that I was Indian, everyone in the class wanted me to be a part of their group for the class project. I remember thinking, "Wow, these kids are so friendly!" When I chose my group, they all looked at me and asked what I thought we should do for the project. I asked what the project was about and realized the topic was Native Americans. Everyone wanted me in their group because they all thought I was Native American Indian! It was an interesting experience, but after I explained the difference, I was glad to become just another student in the class. Thankfully, I was also able to manage quite easily, academically.

Moving to the United States was filled with first experiences. It was so fun to eat new foods like peanut butter and jelly sandwiches and pizza. I remember on our first morning in our new home, my brother and I looked in the cupboards to see what kind of cereal we had. My dad had bought something called "Froot Loops." We ate spoonful after spoonful thinking how it tasted so differently than the Cornflakes we were used to eating. It was so delicious!

Over time, I became a blend of Indian and American culture even though my parents remained the biggest influences in my life. They always emphasized the importance of education and in living your life as a positive force. My mother in particular taught us to treat everyone in our lives with care and kindness. Sadly, she was an uncontrolled diabetic and passed away at 32 due to cardiac complications. I was 13 and my brother was seven years old. It impacted us both deeply and because of her illness, I craved becoming a cardiologist. After finishing up high school at Metro Detroit, I headed to the University of Michigan, where I majored in Biochemistry with the plan to go on to Medical School. I learned along the way though, that life has a way of evolving on its own.

At my university's career day, there was a variety of graduate school booths representing their dental and medical schools. I remember that one of the representatives from the University of Michigan School of Dentistry said that I had a pretty smile, so I went over and chatted with her. The next year, she was back at the career fair and asked me to visit the dental school. Before I knew it, I'd checked it out and was studying for the Dental Admission Test. With her encouragement, I applied to three schools and was fortunate enough to be accepted into all of them. The Dean of each school even called personally to confirm my acceptance! I decided to attend the University of Michigan School of Dentistry. I don't feel that I chose dentistry; it really chose me.

When I graduated in 1991, my personal goals were to work part time and perhaps start a family, since I had married my college sweetheart in my third year of dental school. Life offered another twist, and consequently, our marriage ended after seven years. After the divorce, I moved to Mount Pleasant, where I worked at a very nice family practice. Next, I relocated to the Muskegon area where I entered the public health industry as a dentist. My five years in public health were eye-opening because it allowed me to see the great need for dental services firsthand. However, public health dentists are often limited in the options that we can offer patients—I decided to make the change back to a private practice. That's when I met Jared Van Ittersum, a senior dental student doing an internship at Muskegon Family Care. I observed Jared and really enjoyed the way he treated his patients, not only in terms of his skill set but interpersonally as well. He introduced me to his colleague, Elias Achey, and invited me to visit their practice in Whitehall.

After visiting the Whitehall practice a few times, it became clear that Jared and Elias truly believed in the excellence of dentistry. They embraced higher education, change, and growth. It's not just "drill, fill, and bill" for these guys. Their whole-body approach to dentistry left me feeling like, "Wow this is really cool. These guys have a great idea here!" I knew that I was interested in relating to patients differently. I wanted to involve them as co-therapists, because without their permission, I can't treat them. I wanted to gain the patients' trust and do right by them. I knew that if I achieved that, optimum oral health was possible. I joined Infinity Dental Partners.

Joining this group has been a great experience that has truly nurtured and reinforced my growth as a professional. If I seek additional education, it's encouraged and any time there has been a challenge, both Jared and Elias make the effort to meet with me and we get through it together. They offer me the genuine support that I need to achieve success in my work, while allowing the autonomy of a private practice in terms of how it's run. My philosophy for dentistry is that people are different, they want to be approached differently, treated with respect, and know that they're being heard—Infinity Dental Partners is not here to change that. Even though there is structure and management, there is no pressure to be like the other practices in the partnership.

Within the last year, Infinity Dental Partners has made some changes and, as a result, I've been able to go to the Spring Lake Family Dentistry and start to grow it. It's been a great opportunity. We've made staffing changes that have affected the practice positively and now we have a team of five; including a hygienist, an assistant, one doctor, a team leader, a receptionist, and myself. It's a very cozy practice. After the staff changes, we needed education in team building and conflict resolution techniques and the

Senior Facilitator from Infinity Dental Partners was right there to facilitate the team sessions for us.

I can't stress enough how amazing the management is. If I had come in as a private practitioner taking on Spring Lake Family Dentistry on my own, I would have been doing too many jobs at once. The great thing about being part of Infinity Dental Partners is that they allow me to focus on one thing: dentistry. I don't have to worry about accounting and budgets and management and headaches—Infinity Dental Partners takes those on for me. I trust them because they have proven over time that they are capable of doing a great job. They are organized, focused, and have helped to strengthen our clinical team while growing profits.

It can be easy to take suggestions and changes as interferences, but if you trust the source, you learn to see these changes as things that will benefit the practice overall. I understand that Infinity Dental Partners may have some things figured out that perhaps I don't understand yet. But in order for me to be a good dentist, I need to focus on my job rather than stressing while trying to understand every single step that Infinity Dental Partners takes as a management team. What I've found in the past several months though, is that if something is concerning me, I can quickly text their Senior Facilitator and say, "How do we track this?" He comes back with the answer or he finds someone who will give me the answer. To me, that's a partnership.

Through Infinity Dental Partners, I've been able to attend seminars and trainings that have strengthened me in many ways. When I was part of the Shoreline Dental practice team, we went to a seminar in Fort Lauderdale where Gary Kadi, the educator and author, spoke. During that experience, I learned to eliminate negative thoughts and look at situations in a more positive way. I realized that maybe I should look again at the reasons why I viewed things in a certain light. Another inspiring moment of the conference was learning about the theory of abundance versus the theory of scarcity—it's changed the way I approach life.

To be a good fit for Infinity Dental Partners, you have to trust. If you feel the need to control every single aspect of how a practice is run, then I believe you'll likely have conflict and feel like they are interfering. It's important to relax the reins a bit and take advantage of being part of a practice where you can control the clinical end of it and allow the team to manage the practice. For me, it's a perfect fit.

If you want to grow as a dentist, stay current, and be able to provide quality care that is in tune with current technology, then this is a great place to be. Not only do you have your management needs taken care of, but you also have a network of dentists that you can always connect with, even if it's through Skype or for study clubs to stay in the loop.

I've been a dentist for 20 years now and am so excited to see the ways that dentistry is changing. It's not just about oral care and technology anymore; it's evolving to include both dentists and medical professionals who are expanding the scope of the body/mouth connection in terms of disease control. We are really changing the game by building on this whole-body approach, and Infinity Dental Partners steadily encourages us.

I smile, thinking about how the guys at Infinity Dental Partners see no limit to the possibilities. They serve to empower you and make you feel like you've got wings. That's how they've changed minds.

11

MY BLUE COLLAR ROOTS KEEP ME GROUNDED

by Nicholas C. Ritzema, D.D.S.
Spring Lake, Michigan

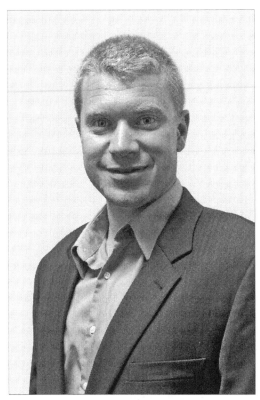

I am originally from a small town north of Grand Rapids, Michigan, called Bailey, which is near Grant. That is where I went to elementary school. Because we lived a good distance from our nearest neighbors, my brothers and I learned to entertain ourselves and appreciate the outdoors. To this day I would much rather be doing something outside than indoors. I have fond memories of helping my parents take care of animals on our farm. Growing up, my father and uncles built the many houses we lived in, so I learned a great deal about construction, such as all the finishes rather than just standard framing. I enjoy home projects and improvements and would love to do more in the future.

I am the oldest of my siblings. I have two younger brothers who are just starting their families and also a sister who is in elementary school. My brothers and I are very close sharing hobbies such as hunting, fishing and sports. I consider them my best friends. My younger sister was born when I was attending college, so although we didn't grow up as close, as my brothers, I still feel I share a unique bond with her. She enjoys staying at my house and playing with my three children.

Prior to middle school, my father built a house in Rockford, and that is where I continued my education and graduated from high school. At Rockford High School I played sports, including track and football. I quickly learned to appreciate and crave an active lifestyle. I met my wife, Krystal, at Rockford, getting to know her through a shared Spanish class. I still can't speak Spanish that well, but am thankful for her willingness to help me and laugh at me, so that I was able to get to know her.

After graduating from high school, I continued my education at Grand Valley State University, earning a degree in Biomedical Sciences. Continuing my love for sports, I participated in their football program, which won several national championships under the leadership of Chuck Martin and Coach Kelly. My positions were outside safety and linebacker. Prior to my acceptance at Grand Valley, the plan was to study mechanical engineering. I quickly learned I was more than capable of doing mechanical engineering, but the workload did not align with the lifestyle I wanted to have. Design and figuring out how things worked appealed to me, yet I wanted to find a career that would allow me to spend quality time with my family. Several family members who are dentists in Northern Michigan inspired me to pursue my career in dentistry. I joined the pre-dental club at GVSU and realized dentistry was "in my blood." My wife also attended GVSU while I was there and we got married one month after graduation.

The year after I graduated from GVSU, I worked for my father's construction company while Krystal and I lived in Sparta. When I applied to dental school, I did not get a position at my first school of choice, which was the University of Michigan, so I was put on the enrollment waiting list. In between work and being a newlywed, I studied hard and re-sat the DAT (Dental Admission Test). I learned of my acceptance that December and was so thankful all of my hard work had paid off.

The following fall, Krystal and I purchased a house on the south side of Brighton after we realized we could afford a house for as much as renting would have been in Ann Arbor. The 2008 housing crisis allowed us to purchase a beautiful three bedroom home that our realtor joked, "When you buy houses with more bedrooms than the number of occupants, you tend to fill the bedrooms up." I laughed and told him there was no way that was going to happen until after I had completed dental school. Well, eleven months later we had our first baby, Grace. The following year we had our second, Kyle. We had two kids in diapers while I was in dental school, so that time in our life was exhausting, but so rewarding at the same time. My wife is a saint. What made it work was that she really held everything together while I studied and helped patients to have healthier mouths. I graduated from Michigan and we moved our family back to West Michigan to be closer to our families. Shortly after moving, we had our last baby, Reese.

I would say the greatest events in my life have been the births of my children, realizing my role as a father, and preparing to emotionally and financially support my family. I am so thankful I've chosen a career in dentistry that allows me to do all of this. Another big event in my life was taking advantage of the housing market crash to put forth the full potential of my money and use it as an investment. Typically when at dental school, a student spends his time at the library with his head in a book, or at the clinic in later years. In addition to doing all of this, I was also thinking, "I have these projects I would like to do with my house so that when I sell it in three or four years, the value will be higher." Outside of dentistry, managing my finances and investment possibilities are things that interest me.

When I was in my last year of dental school, I was introduced to Jared and Elias. As a young dentist, one of the greatest struggles coming out of school was the question, "Where am I going with my dental career?" Thankfully, I had several options graduating dental school and Infinity seemed the most natural fit. Prior to graduating I had researched West Michigan dentists and Infinity was already at the top of my list. I sent my resume to their Spring Lake office and a few days later I received a call from their head of operations, followed by an email. Two weeks later I met Jared and Elias and there was an immediate mutual connection with the outdoors, hunting and salmon fishing. They had a great team, a genuine care for complete health for their patients and an excitement for the future of dentistry that I wanted to be a part of.

From there, everything simply fell into place. I began working with them in a few of their offices four days a week, with the intended goal of working full-time in the Grandville office. Dr. Howell retired from the Grandville office, so I was working there sooner than any of us had anticipated. I appreciate being able to work closer to home, which is now east of Grand Rapids. Working next to Jared allowed me to realize that the way Infinity Dental Partners approach dentistry is also what I envisioned for my dental career. It was a perfect match with regard to their business goals.

In addition to Jared and Elias, my philosophy in dentistry has been influenced by Gary Kadi, our practice consultant. They collaboratively introduced me to complete health dentistry, which I've enjoyed implementing in my own practice.

I spent three days with Gary at a seminar in Detroit, and met many older dentists who were successful, but who were bored. They simply weren't enjoying their profession anymore. The business was frustrating to them and they shared their struggles. At the Gary Kadi meeting, they became enlightened to a new vision of dentistry. I realized what a great opportunity I have, to benefit from this knowledge early on in my career. I approach every day with the vision that I want; helping my patients to be healthy. I enjoy taking time to sit and talk with patients when they come in through our hygiene program. We discuss small and large areas of decay, and large fillings that look good but have the potential to break down in the future. I educate them, so that when there is a disease process occurring in their mouths, they are aware of the potential outcomes and we can evaluate the different treatment options to eliminate the disease process from their bodies. It seems to be something the majority of patients have been reaching out for. They want to know all of their options. This is the information era, where everything is accessible on a cell phone and a solution has been "Googled" or looked up on Web MD. When a patient leaves after being told, "you have tooth decay on number 15" there's a good chance they will leave and Google "tooth decay on number 15" as well as treatment options. I find it best to be honest with patients up front and to educate them with the best route of treatment.

Through my sincerity and honest actions, patients trust I have their utmost care in mind. Some might say I have an old-fashioned approach with patients in that regard, but I enjoy getting to know my patients as well as them getting to know me. This creates a relationship that is beginning to disappear in some practices, but one that I will continue to cherish for years to come. You always hear the story of the old dentist who sat and talked to his patients and knows their whole family and everything about them. I want to be that dentist now and in the future.

I think back to the time I first met Gary Kadi. That event enhanced my vision of what dentistry can and should be, and put me on the trail of educating my patients. I have learned that when they seem perplexed, its not that I've given them too much information, it's that I've given them information they couldn't understand. Oftentimes there is terminology or a procedure that patients are not aware of, and when I take the time to explain, they leave the office feeling confident in me as well as in their treatment. Talking and relating to people is a trait I feel I was naturally born with. I want to know all of my patients and what's going on in their lives. I want to know about their health. I want to be a dentist who can communicate well with their primary care physician, cardiologist, or nurse and effectively answer questions, concerns or problems. The dentist and primary care physician should be the two primary health care directors, and should be able to provide information and point patients in the right direction should they need specialized care.

Having the availability to talk with any of the Infinity Dental Partner dentists has been of immense value to me. I especially get excited when I talk to other dentists in the group about some of the digital aspects, such as CEREC. As far as technology in dentistry goes, I believe the more, the better. Having an open network of communication with a large group of dentists is very advantageous. I have learned many tricks from these dentists who have years of experience, which makes everything easier and faster.

The advice I would give a recent graduate would be to find a practice where you enjoy spending your time and which shares your vision of dentistry. Don't settle for working with someone you wouldn't want to be around seven days a week, let alone the three or four days you actually spend with them. You want to be around someone who shares your vision of dentistry, including how the practice should be run, as well as your outlook on life. If not, there's the possibility of problems, difficulties and struggles.

I see the future of dentistry going towards total health integration and dentists being in communication with primary care physicians and specialists. It seems that many patients over the age of forty have a cardiologist these days. Most patients have a primary care physician, but if not, their dentist may be their only health care provider. I think dentistry has to adapt to work with these health care professionals.

Patients are also becoming more interested in homeopathic treatment. I've had patients come in with a toothache and needing root canal treatment. I'll go over everything with them, educate them, and get them scheduled to come back for the root canal. Then they'll call back and cancel because, at home, they searched on Google and tried to determine what other cheaper forms of treatment are available. They'll come in with stories of putting clove oil on the tooth and it felt so much better that they didn't think they need the root canal anymore. Homeopathic remedies are abundant on the internet, and people are always looking for those. Nobody wants to take medication anymore. Patients need to understand the fact that a homeopathic remedy or a supplement from the GNC store is still a medication. The patient is putting something in his or her body that it doesn't otherwise have. People don't always make the connection that when they're taking a supplement, they basically are taking a medication for symptoms or for an ailment which they have. That's always interesting; trying to be that person who connects the dots between the information that is out there on the internet and what's actually going on with their body. Everybody is different; nobody is the same. That's why an individual approach to treatment is always the best option.

I have to tread lightly sometimes, because there are people who whole-heartedly believe that their information source is absolutely correct, and they'll never disagree with it. I have had patients tell me that fluoride caused problems for them and they don't want to brush their teeth with fluoride toothpaste, yet they want to prevent all these cavities that they keep getting. I have to tell them that fluoride is a natural mineral abundant in well water. It's not just put into city water. They don't like fluoride in their city water, but fluoride is actually put back in the city water after it's removed through the treatment process. Well water has natural fluoride already in it, at different levels depending on where you are in the country, or where you are in the world. Basically, city water is putting it back at an optimum level for it to be healthy for your teeth.

As far as technology in dentistry goes, I believe the more, the better. Patients recognize that we live in a technological world and there are a lot of technologies out there. At some McDonald's, in bigger cities such as Chicago or New York, you order on a touch screen, swipe your credit card and then a server brings out your food. You never actually interact with anyone at the cash register anymore.

Technology in the dental world helps me to interact with my patients in a more positive way. I have the technology to put a digital photograph or digital x-ray up on a large monitor. It's a lot easier to blow it up on a the monitor and then get the patient to look at it and point right at where the disease process is going on and explain the problems to them. Technology in the dental world is making everything easier to diagnose and to explain that diagnosis to patients. That is the biggest benefit.

Patients and dentists alike will definitely have to get used to it and not avoid it. That's where the future of dentistry is headed. Patients are beginning to see the connection between a healthy body and a healthy mouth because all the information is there. Research proves the connection between having a healthy mouth and a healthy body. It's there for people to soak in. If dentistry or certain dentists don't adapt to that, then they're going to fall by the wayside. I'm excited to take an active part in the future of dentistry!

12

RETIREMENT DOESN'T MEAN GOODBYE

by Paul R. Voss, D.D.S.
Whitehall, Michigan

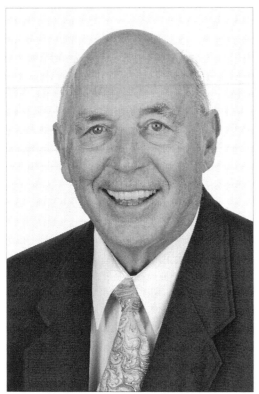

I grew up on Apple Avenue; within the city limits of East Muskegon. At that time, there was a lot of vacant land in the area, and we even had a creek two blocks behind our house. I enjoyed a wonderful childhood that could be described as free-range and easy going. I loved playing sports with the neighborhood kids. We usually played baseball, basketball, or football. The best part was that everyone bent over backwards to allow others to play. If you could stand up, you could play. Nobody was ever left out!

My home life was happy too. My father worked hard so that we were well taken care of. He and I were, and still are, very involved with the church. Both he and my mother were loving, wise, and fair. They encouraged us kids to do our best and to follow our dreams. I had a very good childhood. I feel incredibly fortunate that I was raised the way that I was.

I have one older brother, who I get along with very well. He is three years older than I, and he was an exceptional athlete at school. Both in the classroom and on the field, he was a shining example to me. I also have a sister who is three years younger than me. As is often the case with little sisters, my brother and I always thought she was spoiled, but she grew up to become a well adjusted young lady. She used to work for me for many years, and we still enjoy a strong relationship to this day.

I attended Muskegon High School where I met the girl who became my wife. She and I got married when we were seniors in high school; this interfered; somewhat, with my college plans. It took only half a year of working on a production line at a company named the "Brown Morris Company" to realize that I *had* to further my education. I started out at Muskegon Junior Community College, working towards a degree in chemical engineering. During my time there, I was fortunate enough to get a job with the John Wood Company; a Muskegon Heights manufacturer of gasoline pumps. I worked in the chemical laboratory, all the while juggling my studies with making time for my wife and our growing family. Even though I was going to school part-time and working part-time, having this job at the pumps gave me a taste of what chemical engineering work entailed. I soon discovered that it wasn't for me. I felt too isolated from other people. The particular position I held did not compel me to continue along the course of study I was, at that time, on.

During that time, my wife and I had a serious discussion about career choices, and I mentioned that I had always had a desire to enter into the field of medicine in some capacity. Feeling inspired by this new possibility, I visited a number of physicians and dentists and asked them about their careers. One physician told me, "As a physician, I make a wonderful living. But I do it for my family, not for myself. I'm too busy to have much time for myself." Every dentist I talked to, on the other hand, loved what they did and were happy with the hours. They also made a reasonable living and provided well for their families.

Consequently, I decided to pursue a career within the field of dentistry. As I finished community college, I applied to attend the University of Michigan Dental School. When I found out that I had been shortlisted I telephoned the Dean to request an interview with him. He responded affirmatively, so I went to Ann Arbor and we talked for an hour and a half. At the end of our discussion I asked him whether or not I had made it to the admissions. Noncommittally, he said, "We'll let you know." My frustrated reply was, "I really need to know now!"

At that time, I had two children, and my wife was willing to work. I told the Dean I had to find lodging near the university for myself and a house for my family in Ann Arbor, and make arrangements for a move, because it was going to take me five years to get through two years worth of school while working. I emphasized yet again that I really needed to know whether I should be applying elsewhere. After some hesitation, he said, "Well, you're in." Immediately after the interview, I made arrangements for housing and accommodation for our family in Ann Arbor, and my wife got a job in that area.

I was very fortunate to get into dental school after attending community college for only two years. I was told that I was not supposed to work while attending dental school, but I didn't have much of a choice. So I took care of mice, rabbits, and other animals at the medical school's medical center. After that, I drove a bus for a while. The best job I had during that time was with a company called Conductor Inc.. I became the company liaison and courier, I also spent time working in the security department. I was able to stay with that company for about four years.

I was granted approval to take a year off from school between my sophomore and junior years so I could earn more money. I remained with Conductor, Inc. until I graduated from dental school in 1966, a full decade after my graduation from high school. Then I worked in Ann Arbor for three months, waiting for my kids to finish their schooling, and waiting for the necessary arrangements to be made for a move to Whitehall, Michigan, where I had purchased a practice from a dentist.

The doctor from whom I had purchased the practice was retiring. Although he retired in May, I was unable to start my career, due to certain circumstances, until early in July. For the first time in what seemed like forever, I actually had some time to myself! I went fishing on the Upper Peninsula for about three weeks. Then, on July 5, 1966, I started my own practice in Whitehall.

I will have to say that the greatest influence in my life while growing up was The Church and Jesus Christ. My love for Jesus continued into adulthood and became the foundation of who I am as an individual and guided me as to how I was going to raise my family and conduct my life.

My wife and I have two daughters. One lives in Montague, where I also live. Our other daughter lives in Long Beach, California. We are fortunate to have plenty of contact with them both. We also have four grandchildren. Our eldest granddaughter lives and works in Dallas and our other granddaughter lives and works in New York City. One grandson has just graduated from the

University of Michigan and is now working in Ann Arbor. Our other grandson on the West Coast is currently a senior at the University of Southern California. Although the kids are scattered around the country, I am blessed in my ability to maintain good contact with them and to see them as often as I can.

I am quite content with life at the moment, even though I was diagnosed with multiple myeloma in 2005. This was a terminal cancer that had grown unexpectedly and aggressively. Blessedly, I was given the opportunity to participate in a clinical trial at the University of Michigan, which has worked wonders for me. The disease is still present, but it seems to be under control. I still undergo chemotherapy every day, although the trial itself, which involved the infusion of caustic drugs into my system, ended in November 2011.

With regards to my health, I've been holding my own ever since, notwithstanding one brief period of relapse. Tragically, as soon as we had received the good news that the clinical trial was ending, my wife unexpectedly passed away. This was in December 2011. Her passing radically altered the plans we had made together. My world was shaken, and my outlook on life had completely changed. Still, I knew that I had been blessed to have spent 56 wonderful years with my high school sweetheart, and although I miss Marilyn every day, life has still been good to me. I feel well. I do my best to stay active. I volunteer at various places and lead a pleasant life with plenty of friends by my side. Altogether, things are going well for me.

In addition to my marriage to Marilyn and our two beautiful daughters, dental school itself was another major factor in my life, and the fact that I was able to attend after completing only two years of college education is something that I will always be thankful for. The births of my grandchildren were also wonderful events. My family was, and always will be, extremely important to me. My dad lived to become 104 years old, and my mom reached the age of 99, so I was very fortunate to have had them around a lot. They played a large part in helping me become the man I am today.

When sharing advice or expressing my outlook to others, I will always say that developing a spiritual life is incredibly important; that is the single best advice I can impart. I believe that it's very important to have a strong faith in Jesus Christ. This is something that I have discussed at length with my grandchildren. Although I sometimes wish to see more progress in them, I rest, assured that they respect my advice and are living decent lives. I do my best to walk with honesty and integrity. I believe in something that transcends the Golden Rule, that you should treat people in a manner that is better than the manner in which you expect to be treated. That has long been my motto, and throughout my life, following this advice has provided significant dividends, long-lasting friendships, and beneficial associations.

Joining Infinity was, in my estimation, one of the highlights in my life, although it seemed to come out of the blue. I was, as I mentioned, diagnosed with terminal cancer in 2005, and I couldn't physically keep up with the workload involved in running an individual practice anymore. I continued to work as I went through chemo but, in 2006, I did bring in an associate with the understanding that she was eventually going to take over the practice. Although she was supposed to purchase the practice by 2008, she seemed rather reluctant to take that step. I patiently continued with the arrangement we had in place, but she never seemed in any hurry to take over the practice, nor did I receive any viable explanation as to why.

Then one day, in mid-November 2010, Bob Burton from Echo called me and said that Elias and Jared were interested in purchasing my practice. My reply was, "Bob, your timing is kind of bad because I will be leaving tomorrow for California." Undaunted, he answered, "Call me when you get back." My wife and I spent two weeks in California over Thanksgiving and discussed this possibility while we were there. When we got back in early December, I contacted Bob and said,

"Let's find out what's going on." Bob reiterated that Elias and Jared would like to complete the purchase by the end of the year, if possible.

Even though December was a busy time with the Christmas holidays, both parties managed to negotiate an offer by the end of the month. My associate was informed of the situation, and the plan went through on December 31, 2010. Ever since, I have been enjoying a wonderful relationship with Infinity, as well as with Elias and Jared. I couldn't be happier with my current situation. Working for Infinity Dental Partners has really been a relief, especially since the passing of my wife.

This opportunity turned out to be a blessing beyond belief. Without the added responsibility of running a practice, I was able to find more time for myself and able to focus on my own health. After working with Infinity Dental Partners for some time, I chose to retire completely. However, Infinity Dental Partners continues to include me in some of their events so I still feel that I am part of the team. In fact, I hope to participate once again in Infinity's free dental day in 2014. This has been the greatest working relationship I could ask for. I personally don't believe that I could have found a situation that would be more ideal for me, and I can only hope that my colleagues feel the same way!

My association with Infinity Dental Partners relieved me of much stress. The difference Infinity has made to my life is very significant. They took over all the management, scheduling, and personnel, so that during my time with them, all I had to do was work; treating patients was the part of dentistry that I loved the most anyway. The Infinity Dental Partners staff has treated me with more respect than I probably deserve. At the age of 75, they view me as a type of grandfather figure, which I enjoy. Since my retirement, Jared, Elias, and the staff at Infinity have maintained close ties with me. When we are together, I truly feel like a member of the Infinity family. In fact, I feel as if I have passed my business over to a son, rather than a mere purchaser. My closeness with the staff continues to this day. As a case in point, I stopped in at the Whitehall practice the other day and Elias happened to be there. He came over and gave me a big hug and a happy greeting, and we were able to have a chat and catch up. I can't even express to you the dimension and joy that Infinity has added to my life.

The situation at Infinity Dental Partners has worked out beautifully because both my daughter and son-in-law are chiropractors in Whitehall, and we were sharing our building with them for a time. When they decided they wanted more room for their practice, the staff at Infinity Dental Partners moved to the pre-existing White Lake Family Dentistry building, which turned out perfectly for all involved. The transition of employees was very smooth, in my opinion, although several of them chose to move to other practices.

As far as I know, the Infinity patients have accepted the transition very well. Needless to say, there are a few that haven't, but a large number seem to feel very comfortable with the situation. When I was practicing on my own, I spent a lot of time talking with patients, who came to become like family and friends to me. I have found that this still seems to still be the case with Infinity Dental Partners at the White Lake Family Dentistry. Patients are still treated as friends, and a family-type atmosphere still exists. Even though it's on a larger scale, it is still a rather small town practice. People are treated and cared for as individuals. For the most part, everyone is very happy.

When talking to a few people who were considering joining Infinity Dental Partners, my advice was, "This is a situation that seems too good to be true, but it is true. I personally couldn't be happier." To anyone who's thinking of joining, I would say, "Absolutely, yes!" Infinity Dental Partners has done everything they have said they would do and then some in order to make this arrangement work comfortably for me. I know that they have a business to run, and that their interests come first, but I think that they have also made me a high priority when it comes to their decisions and considering my requests.

This continued even after the merger, when we were all working together; if, for instance, I wanted to use a different laboratory, they would say, "Go ahead and do it; do your own thing." Therefore, I was still part of the team, but was able to act independently with regards to some of the things that I wanted. As I've told a number of people, "It's too good to be true, but it is true."

I had a high degree of autonomy from the standpoint that I could continue planning treatments and scheduling my hours the way I wanted to. I never felt as if "Big Brother" were standing over my shoulder and saying, "You need to do it this way," or, "You need to work these hours." The company has always been more than supportive of my rights as an individual, as well as a team member. We often participated in various talks and get-togethers in order to discuss different components of the practice and its procedures. They were very understanding about what I wanted, and were continually supportive of my particular needs.

While the future of dentistry depends on our government, dentistry is still an exciting field to pursue. It is the only area of medicine that actively strives to put itself out of a job by stressing the preventive aspects of dental care.

Infinity Dental Partners dentists do a very remarkable job of this. Group practices with strong associations like this are extremely viable, as well as being better able to afford expensive dental equipment and perform a quality dental service. Although dentistry itself is a healthy industry, one who chooses to go it alone is likely to fall behind with regard to technology. One or two people in a practice can't do what a group can do. To my way of thinking, a strong group practice is the way to go.

31704543R00133

Made in the USA
Charleston, SC
25 July 2014